HIV/AIDS, stigma and child....

A literature review

Harriet Deacon and Inez Stephney

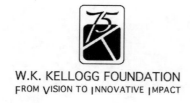

W.K. KELLOGG FOUNDATION
FROM VISION TO INNOVATIVE IMPACT

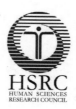

HSRC
HUMAN SCIENCES
RESEARCH COUNCIL

Published by HSRC Press
Private Bag X9182, Cape Town, 8000, South Africa
www.hsrcpress.ac.za

First published 2007

ISBN 978-0-7969-2188-8

© 2007 Human Sciences Research Council

Copyedited by Vaun Cornell
Typeset by Janco Yspeert
Cover design by Oryx Media
Cover photo: ©Branko de Lang/iAfrika Photos
Print management by Compress

Distributed in Africa by Blue Weaver
Tel: +27 (0) 21 701 4477; Fax: +27 (0) 21 701 7302
www.oneworldbooks.com

Distributed in Europe and the United Kingdom by Eurospan Distribution Services (EDS)
Tel: +44 (0) 20 7240 0856; Fax: +44 (0) 20 7379 0609
www.eurospangroup.com/bookstore

Distributed in North America by Independent Publishers Group (IPG)
Call toll-free: (800) 888 4741; Fax: +1 (312) 337 5985
www.ipgbook.com

CONTENTS

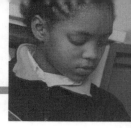

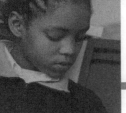

ACKNOWLEDGEMENTS

The literature review has benefited from comments by various people to whom we are most grateful. Thanks go specifically to Donald Skinner, Lucie Cluver, Bendan Maugham-Brown, Lauren Wild, and Helen Meintjes for comments on the paper.

ACRONYMS AND ABBREVIATIONS

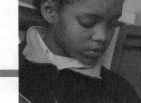

CABA	children affected by HIV/AIDS
CAPS	Cape Area Panel Study
CAS	Cape Area Study
CRC	(UN) Convention on the Rights of the Child
CSSR	Cenre for Social Science Research
NGO	non-governmental organisation
KAB	knowledge-attitudes-behaviours
OVC	orphans and vulnerable children
PLWHA	people living with HIV/AIDS
SAHARA	Social Aspects of HIV/AIDS Research Alliance

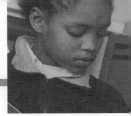

CHAPTER I

Introduction

1.1   Children and the HIV/AIDS pandemic

The UN Convention on the Rights of the Child (CRC) states that children are 'entitled to special care and assistance' and that this care and assistance should enable 'full and harmonious development' (CRC in Amon 2002: 143). There is a general consensus that there is an onus on society in general to care for children (especially when family care is inadequate), and that negative experiences in childhood can have very long-term effects on adults, and thus on the future of a society.

The HIV/AIDS pandemic poses major threats to the socio-economic and psychological welfare of HIV-affected and infected children. The pandemic can adversely affect household stability and sustainability, children's access to healthcare and schooling, state of health and nutrition, and increase affected children's vulnerability to infection (Richter et al. 2004). It can also increase the extent to which children are placed prematurely in the position of caregivers and household heads (Barrett et al. 1999; Stein et al. 1999).

The massive impact of the HIV/AIDS pandemic on children and their support systems in families and communities has prompted fears that millions of children will not receive proper care and assistance for their proper development (Amon 2002). While these fears have prompted increased research interest in children affected by HIV/AIDS, a number of researchers now suggest that concerns about threats to state security posed by growing numbers of orphans have been overstated – the main challenge is addressing increased poverty in high-prevalence countries (Nattrass 2002). Extended family support systems have mitigated or delayed the effects of widespread orphanhood on society (Gilborn et al. 2001). Children of migrant workers have historically experienced similar disadvantages to those affected by HIV/AIDS in sub-Saharan Africa, and children affected by HIV/AIDS are more likely to become depressed than to act out their distress (Bray 2003; Poulter 1997; Wild et al. 2005).

A large number of organisations have attempted specifically to address the needs of children in the context of HIV/AIDS. Most concern about assessing and addressing the needs of HIV-affected children initially focused on identifying material needs that would no longer be met in conditions of increasing poverty, absence of parental protection and the erosion of existing support and educational systems in the HIV/AIDS pandemic (Ali 1998; Gilborn et al. 2001; Segu & Wolde-Yohannes 2000). There has been some recent attention paid to the psychological needs of children affected by HIV/AIDS, a discussion in which stigma has featured prominently (see for example, Daniel 2005; Foster et al. 1997; Foster & Williamson 2000; Fox 2002; Geballe et al. 1995; Siegel & Gorey 1994).

1.2   Children and HIV/AIDS-related stigma

HIV/AIDS-related stigma has been recognised as a key problem that needs to be addressed in HIV/AIDS interventions with adults (for a review, see Deacon et al. 2005). The literature on children and HIV/AIDS is extensive, as is the literature on HIV/AIDS-related stigma, but specific research on HIV/AIDS-related stigma and children is relatively sparse.

This research suggests that stigma and discrimination can exacerbate the material and psychological problems children already face in the context of the HIV/AIDS pandemic (Chase & Aggleton 2001; Clay et al. 2003; Geballe et al. 1995; Gernholtz & Richter 2004). Stigma can prevent proper access to education, well-being, treatment and care both directly (through abuse, denial of care, forced child labour and loss of inheritance), and indirectly (if children avoid potentially stigmatising situations such as social interaction, healthcare and educational opportunities because they expect or internalise stigma) (Strode & Barrett-Grant 2001). Stigma, discrimination and courtesy stigma directed towards adults can affect the ability of caregivers to provide proper psychosocial and material support for children infected or affected by HIV/AIDS (Juma et al. 2004; Robertson & Ensink 1992).

Research on adults cannot be extrapolated directly to children because children are likely to be affected by stigma and discrimination in different ways from adults. Children are developing cognitively, physically and socially, and they may interpret, express and react to stigma in different ways from adults. Because children are particularly vulnerable to courtesy stigma (for example, that associated with parental HIV status), they might experience stigma more intensely than adults do (Cree et al. 2004). Children may also be more vulnerable to discrimination because they are often not in as much control of their circumstances as are adults, they often do not know their rights, and may be less able to assert their rights.

There is variation in the extent, effects, and nature of stigma and discrimination across regional, cultural, socio-economic and gender contexts. Stigma and discrimination can be affected by various epidemiological factors including stage of the epidemic, prevalence, distribution of HIV cases, political factors and so on (Deacon et al. 2005). While this variation does not always imply the need for different interventions to reduce stigma (Ogden & Nyblade 2005), it does suggest that research on children in other contexts may not be directly applicable in sub-Saharan Africa, and even within the region there may be significant differences in children's experiences.

In spite of ample anecdotal and descriptive evidence that HIV/AIDS-related stigma and discrimination are affecting children, not enough systematic research has been done to illustrate the nature and extent of the problem, and how it relates to other key sources of disadvantage for children in poor, high-prevalence areas. Addressing the needs of children affected by HIV/AIDS is particularly important in developing countries, not only because the proportion of young people in these societies is very high (about 32 per cent of South Africans are under 15 years of age, for example [Stats SA 2005: 11]), but because young people are at high risk of contracting HIV.

This paper reviews the literature on HIV/AIDS, children and stigma to interrogate the following questions:
- What is the evidence that HIV/AIDS-related stigma and discrimination directly affects children, both materially and psychologically?
- How does HIV/AIDS-related stigma impact (materially and psychologically) on adult caregivers and household structures supporting children affected by HIV/AIDS?
- How is HIV/AIDS-related stigma articulated in relation to children in different social, economic and cultural contexts?
- What role do children play in the process of stigmatisation itself? Do children stigmatise other children more than, or in different ways from, adults?

- Are there different developmental impacts on (and responses to) stigma depending on the age of the child? If so, how is this related to emotional or cognitive development?

1.3   Methodology

The purpose of this kind of literature review is intentionally somewhat broader than a brief review of key studies often used to summarise theoretical positions or justify decisions taken in a particular research project. The paucity of literature specifically on children, HIV/AIDS and stigma has influenced the approach we have taken. In this review we aim to:

- Understand some of the underlying factors that have driven certain kinds of inquiry and debate in the field of research on children and HIV/AIDS;
- Analyse what has been written on the topic of children and HIV/AIDS-related stigma;
- Determine what can be learned from comparative research on other forms of stigma or work on child development;
- Make recommendations on broad research questions or hypotheses, methodological approaches, data analysis and interventions in the field as a whole.

A bibliographic database was developed in Reference Manager by Inez Stephney and Alison Bullen. The database included published and unpublished studies on children and disease-related stigma and on the effects of the HIV/AIDS pandemic on children, including the literature on orphans and vulnerable children. Searches were done on various databases on EBSCO Host including Academic Premier, MasterFILE Premier, Health Source, Medline, PsycINFO and PsycARTICLES, and on Google and Google Scholar. Key non-governmental organisation (NGO) websites were accessed for additional grey literature.

The database of bibliographic references generated in this project was added to a larger Reference Manager database on disease-related stigma developed for a previous literature review on stigma and adults (Deacon et al. 2005). Copies of the entire database will be made available during 2006 on the SAHARA website.[1]

Harriet Deacon led the writing of the review paper, to which Inez Stephney made contributions in the sections on effects of the pandemic on support systems and on the content of stigma. Analysis of the literature was conducted after reading abstracts and articles, and creating subsets of the database on issues such as disclosure, bereavement and knowledge acquisition. We have looked primarily at research on adolescents (10–18 years) and young children (approximately 5–10 years). The most useful comparative material was found in research on children and epilepsy stigma.

Having explained what we plan to do in this study, we will now briefly define some key concepts in Chapter 2. The literature review itself will be covered in Chapter 3. Recommendations for research and interventions are discussed in Chapter 4 and we conclude the study in Chapter 5.

---

1 www.sahara.org.za

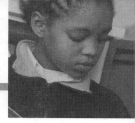

CHAPTER 2

Definitions

2.1   Defining stigma

In the last few years the introduction of ideas from critical social theory, both from social psychology and from disciplines like sociology, has occasioned something of a debate about theory and method in stigma research, which has in the past been dominated by attitudinal studies in psychology.

This debate suggests, firstly, that we need to challenge the 'conceptual inflation' of stigma. The concept of stigma seems endlessly elastic, an idea that has so much scope it cannot hold its core (see Stafford & Scott 1986 cited in Weiss & Ramakrishna 2001). As one paper commented:

> Stigma...is creaking under the burden of explaining a series of disparate, complex and unrelated processes to such an extent that use of the term is in danger of obscuring as much as it enlightens. (Prior et al. 2003: 128)

Secondly, we need to define stigma more clearly. Many researchers have bemoaned the lack of a common theoretical perspective on stigma (Link & Phelan 2001), and there has been some work done towards better theoretical perspectives (Deacon et al. 2005; Joffe 1999; Parker & Aggleton 2003). Much of the research on stigma has conflated stigmatising beliefs themselves (unjustified negative things people believe about others that involve a moral judgement), responses to stigma (internalisation of negative beliefs, or expected stigma and discrimination), and effects of stigma like discrimination (what people do to disadvantage others).

Because unfair discrimination is one of the main reasons why stigma is a problem, many studies define stigma as something that results in discrimination, suggesting that discrimination is the enactment or end point of stigma (for example, Link & Phelan 2001). This position has come out of the tradition of understanding stigma research as a way of identifying and tackling human rights issues in HIV and AIDS work. Thus, work like Parker and Aggleton (2003), for example, emphasises the way in which stigma and discrimination follow the fault-lines of existing social marginalisation. This links to a broader effort to link HIV prevention to poverty relief and improvement in women and children's rights.

Poverty relief and human rights activism are laudable causes, and should continue to be priorities on their own merits, but the above approach is not necessarily the best model for understanding and researching stigma. Stigma and discrimination are not inextricably intertwined in practice, since not all stigmatising beliefs lead to discrimination and not all discrimination is due to stigma. Stigma is just one possible cause of disadvantage. Castro and Farmer (2005) for example, argue that stigma is less important than logistical and economic barriers to health service access in Haiti. It is not easy to determine to what extent stigma specifically contributes to the intensification and reproduction of social inequalities, because even without stigmatisation, marginalised people would be more likely to contract HIV and the HIV/AIDS pandemic would exacerbate existing inequalities (Heywood 2002).

Also, stigma can have serious negative effects without resulting in unfair discrimination, for example, when people who are stigmatised avoid social encounters because they fear status loss or discrimination as a result of such encounters. Defining stigma as something that always leads to discrimination downplays the very real impact stigmatising beliefs may have on the self-concept and actions of stigmatised people in the absence of any active discrimination against them.

The relationship between stigma and existing forms of disadvantage is structurally, ideologically and conceptually complex. Understanding stigma and discrimination mainly as processes that only target those who are already marginalised is useful only in the broadest sense – the process linking stigma and disadvantage is much more complex, and the solutions we must seek to both problems are also much more complex.

Following the work of Miles (1989) on racism, Deacon et al. (2005) therefore suggest analytically separating the *ideology* of stigma from *responses* to stigma and the *effects* of stigma (such as the practice of unfair discrimination). This allows researchers to explore knowledge, attitudes, internalisation and unfair practices without necessarily assuming they are all in a one-to-one relationship. We also define stigma as a blaming and othering response, a cognitive justification for an emotional reaction of fear. Stigma allows people to distance themselves from the risk of infection by blaming contraction of the disease on characteristics normally associated with outgroups. Health-related stigmatisation is an ideology formulated through the following social process:
1. Constructing illness as preventable or controllable;
2. Identifying 'immoral' behaviours causing the disease;
3. Associating these behaviours with 'carriers' of the disease in other groups; and
4. Thus blaming certain people for their own infection; and
5. Justifying (although not necessarily engaging in) discrimination against them. (Joffe 1999 adapted in Deacon et al. 2005).

It is also worth defining other aspects of stigma. Secondary stigma can be defined as stigma attached to other things (diseases, objects and practices) because of their association with HIV/AIDS, for example formula feeding or tuberculosis in the South African context. Courtesy stigma is stigma attached to people because of their association with HIV/AIDS or HIV-positive people, for example stigmatisation of family members of a person identified as having HIV/AIDS, or stigmatisation of healthcare workers who work with people living with HIV/AIDS (PLWHA).

Stigmatised people's responses to stigma can include self-stigmatisation (i.e. internalisation of stigma), for example when PLWHA come to agree with the social perception of themselves as devalued, and perceived or expected stigma and discrimination, for example when PLWHA make decisions based on a judgement of the likely stigmatising or discriminatory consequences for them.

These definitions allows us to explore in greater detail the relationship between stigma and ignorance, existing forms of prejudice, marginalisation and disadvantage, negative associations with sexuality and death, and forms of social interaction such as rumour and gossip. These issues will be discussed in greater detail in the review, but we wish to make a few preliminary comments about the concept of layered stigma.

2.2   Layered stigma

We have argued above that the process of 'othering' draws on existing patterns of social differentiation:

> Categories of blame often reflect deep social-class biases. Illness is frequently associated with poverty and becomes a justification for social inequities... disease is frequently associated with the 'other', be it the other race, the other class, the other ethnic group. Inevitably the locus of blame is also tied to specific ideological, political and social concerns. (Nelkin & Gilman 1988)

> Diseases from hookworm to tuberculosis to cancer, polio, sickle cell anemia and AIDS have been employed as markers of biological and social difference, and also to construct broader notions of danger and inferiority. (Wailoo 2001)

The notion of layered stigma borrows from the notion of double or triple oppression used in debates about women's rights. It suggests that stigma follows the fault-lines of society and, in Africa, deepens existing social divisions between men and women, rich and poor, white and black. The poor are both more vulnerable to HIV/AIDS, more likely to suffer its effects publicly at a household and personal level, and more vulnerable to discrimination (Ogden & Nyblade 2005). As Joffe (1999) has suggested, however, the process of stigmatisation is not just a replication of existing power relations. Poorer groups can stigmatise wealthier and more powerful groups too, both within and between societies: Africans, for example, can blame western science and western immorality for creating and spreading HIV. It is of course true that stigmatisation of the powerful often has no effect on them (Link & Phelan 2006). At a global level, HIV/AIDS-related stigma has been stronger and discrimination has been more intense against marginalised groups like gay men, women, poor people, Africans, drug users, Haitians and African Americans.

But although discrimination may affect higher status members of society less, stigmatisation does nevertheless affect them. People in the middle classes may experience more obvious status anxiety than people in lower or upper socio-economic groups (Fox 2004). In a western context, wealthy people and heterosexuals might experience greater status loss if they contract HIV/AIDS because they do not fit with the risk categories of inner-city drug users or gay men in the layered stigmatising discourse (see also Ogden & Nyblade 2005), but they may be able to hide their status or weather the consequences of discrimination better.

In areas of greater poverty and a generalised HIV/AIDS epidemic, more blame can be directed at high status members of a society if their HIV status becomes known because they have more social status to lose, and 'should have known better' (Bond et al. 2003). Thus, if the priest gets HIV it may be more difficult to for him to disclose his HIV-positive status because it results in greater status loss than if, say a sex worker discloses her status. Wealth often provides the ability to keep stigmatising information secret, perhaps by visiting private rather than public health facilities, or getting treatment early. People wealthy enough to send their child away if that child is pregnant or has HIV are wealthy enough to avoid loss of social status in their community, but they also thereby lose access to their child and have to bear the secret al.one. The consequences of stigmatisation are thus different, but may be no less intense, for high status members of a society.

HIV/AIDS-related stigma is not just replicating existing forms of social marginalisation or structural disadvantage such as poverty, but it is interacting with other exclusionary discourses and practices (such as sexism for example) that may cut across these categories. Different forms of social stigmatisation or exclusion may thus affect someone, even where these forms of social stigma or disadvantage are not necessarily linked. Link and Phelan (2006) suggest that the full effects of stigmatisation and related discrimination are not fully recognised by researchers because attempts to measure the impact of stigma have generally restricted analysis to one circumstance (e.g. AIDS, obesity, race, or mental illness) and examined only one outcome (e.g. earnings, self esteem, housing, or social interactions). If all stigmatised conditions were considered together and all outcomes examined we believe that stigma would be shown to have an enormous impact on people's lives. To exemplify one part of this point we analysed nationally representative data from the USA, in which multiple stigmatising factors were taken into consideration in relation to self-esteem, and found that stigma could explain a full 20 per cent of the variance beyond the effects of age, sex, and years of education.

In conclusion, we have developed a definition of stigma that distinguishes between stigma as ideology and discrimination as practice, and notes the lack of a one-to-one relationship between the two. In order to address stigma we need to understand the effects of stigma better (these can include status loss, related discrimination, internalisation, and social withdrawal). We also need to understand the relationships between various kinds of stigma and existing forms of marginalisation or disadvantage. These relationships are complex and sometimes cumulative, and can seriously reduce quality of life in infected or affected people.

2.3   Defining 'children'

In this paper we subscribe to the following broad view of childhood adopted by sociologists of childhood, the CRC and other rights-based approaches to development:
(a)   Childhood is not a homogenous state, and differs cross-culturally;
(b)   Children are significantly differentiated through factors such as age, gender, or ethnicity;
(c)   Children are social actors who engage in and have effects on the social world around them; and
(d)   Children have rights and opinions and should therefore participate in determining what happens to them. (West & Wedgwood 2004)

In writing this literature review, we are interested in developing a general framework for conducting research on AIDS-related stigma and children, so we have tried to draw on a wide range of the literature on children and HIV/AIDS. Much of the research on children and HIV/AIDS tends to focus on specific categories of children who are at risk for adverse effects and/or contraction of HIV. These categories include orphans, adolescents, HIV-negative children of HIV-positive parents, HIV-positive children, inner-city African-American children, and poor African children.

These children may have different experiences of HIV/AIDS and stigma, but there are also commonalities and overlaps between categories, as can be seen in Figure 1, with the categories 'orphans', 'street children' and 'children living with HIV/AIDS'. We need a better understanding of differences and commonalities relevant to research on HIV/AIDS-related stigma and children. In this review we have therefore tried to range across the various existing categories in order to create a framework for cutting the conceptual cake in new ways if necessary. We have therefore made use of the general category 'children', where we feel that findings can be generalised.

Figure 1: Children from stigmatised groups

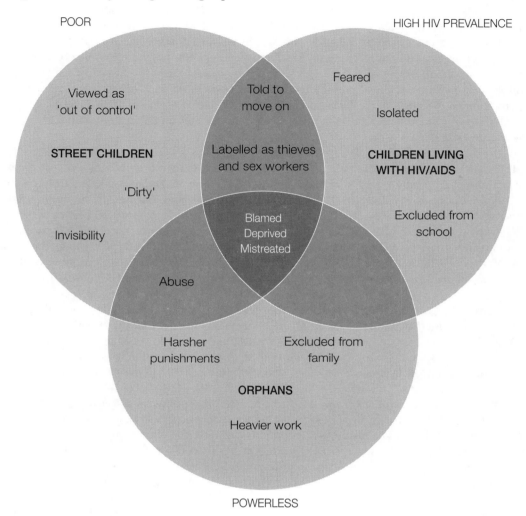

POOR

HIGH HIV PREVALENCE

Viewed as
'out of control'

Told to
move on

Feared

Isolated

STREET CHILDREN

Labelled as thieves
and sex workers

**CHILDREN LIVING
WITH HIV/AIDS**

'Dirty'

Blamed
Deprived
Mistreated

Excluded from
school

Invisibility

Abuse

Harsher
punishments

Excluded from
family

ORPHANS

Heavier work

POWERLESS

Source: Clay et al. 2003: 20

In this study, we have looked primarily at research on adolescents (11–18 years) and young children (approximately 5–10 years), although the likelihood of HIV/AIDS-related stigma having some negative effects on newborns and very small children is noted. Although opinions differ as to when childhood actually ends (the cut-off point ranging from 15 to 21), it is generally understood as 'a period of rapid growth and development' after birth in which a child matures both physically and psychologically 'in ways that define intellectual, social, spiritual, and emotional characteristics' for adult life (Amon 2002: 143).

UNICEF and UNAIDS initially defined children as 15 years and under (UNCR & UNAIDS 2000 cited in Abebe 2005), but this has been increased to 18 years and under (UNAIDS et al. 2004) to come into line with the CRC. Skinner et al. (2004) suggest that community definitions of childhood in Africa include children up to the age of 18, an idea already enshrined in the African Union's 1999 African Charter on the Rights and Welfare of the Child.

Interestingly, the definition of adolescence seems to extend beyond most of the standard end points for childhood. It seems to be a category defined largely by entry into puberty and sexual activity. The American Centers for Disease Control (CDC) define adolescence from age 10 to 24, while the WHO defines adolescence from 10 to 19 years. The psychological literature generally distinguishes between early adolescence (10–13 years), middle adolescence (14–16 years) and late adolescence (17–20 years). Thus, a late adolescent in some of the stigma literature might be defined as a young adult by African communities (Skinner et al. 2004) and as an adult in the UNAIDS or UNICEF data. This underlines the need for careful attention to be paid to age ranges in the comparative literature on stigma.

Most data on orphans in the past referred to children less than 15 years old, but in recent years more frequently refers to children under 18 (Grassly & Timaeus 2003). Orphans are generally understood – both in the international literature and among African communities and service providers – as children who have lost at least one parent (Skinner et al. 2004). Not all orphans have lost both biological parents, therefore. Maternal and paternal orphans have respectively lost their mother and father only, and double orphans have lost both parents. The Actuarial Society of South Africa (ASSA) models include double orphans in their calculations for both maternal and paternal orphans (Meintjes & Giese 2006).

The term 'AIDS orphan' has been coined to refer specifically to that category of children who are orphaned by parental AIDS. An AIDS orphan is thus defined by UNAIDS as 'a child who has at least one parent dead from AIDS' and a double (or dual) AIDS orphan as 'a child whose mother and father have both died, at least one due to AIDS' (UNAIDS Reference Group on Estimates Modelling and Projections 2002 in Grassly & Timaeus 2003).

Many researchers comment on the need to understand orphans as a socially constructed category: in Malawi, for example, social definitions of orphanhood emphasise loss and need, allowing the inclusion of older people as orphans and the exclusion of some children who have been successfully fostered or adopted (Chirwa 2002). Meintjes and Giese (2006) argue that South African community definitions of orphanhood refer to the inability of parents to provide for their children, so children of poor parents may be described as 'orphans' (at least in translation) and well-provided-for children with no parents may not be described as orphans. Imposing external definitions of orphanhood on children may be stigmatising.

In Uganda, Ntozi and Mukiza-Gapere (1995) show how social definitions of orphanhood have changed as a consequence of the HIV/AIDS epidemic: in the past, children who lost one parent would not be considered orphans as it was common practice for their remaining parent to remarry. The increased likelihood that both parents have HIV/AIDS, fear that the remaining parent is HIV-positive, stigmatisation of widows as witches (see also Mukumbira 2002), and the impoverishment of AIDS-affected households has resulted in fewer remaining parents remarrying (even if they are HIV-negative).

The term 'orphans and vulnerable children' (OVC) was coined to extend the discussion of disadvantage beyond orphans to other categories of children (for example, children of sick parents). Vulnerability is also socially defined (Skinner et al. 2004; Smart 2003), and creating an overarching definition is therefore difficult (Skinner et al. 2004, Foster & Williamson 2000; Monk 2002 in Grassly & Timaeus 2003). Grassly and Timaeus suggest that creating a single definition of OVC 'is unnecessary, so long as there is some attempt to quantify this indirect effect of HIV on child welfare' (2003: 3). Indeed, they say, 'the definition of a vulnerable child is more often determined by data availability than conceptual issues' (UNICEF and UNAIDS 2003 in Grassly & Timaeus 2003: 3).

Giese et al. (2003b) suggest a reasonable compromise definition of OVC as follows: 'those whose care is compromised as a result of the terminal illness or death of an adult who contributes substantially to the care and/or financial support of the child'. However, this definition underplays the extent to which children may be impacted by the death or illness of siblings or peers.[2]

The needs of each child will depend on the interaction of various factors (for example, poverty, death of caregiver) and how the child copes with them in a specific environment. The impact of certain circumstances (e.g. orphanhood) will change over the course of the epidemic or the child's life as cumulative effects increase (for example, as more alternative caregivers die, the impact on remaining healthy households is greater). There are thus varying levels of vulnerability (Skinner et al. 2004). Skinner et al. (2004) suggest key variables determining vulnerability include: material problems (access to money, food, clothing, shelter, healthcare and education); emotional problems (including experience of caring, love, support, space to grieve and containment of emotions); and social problems (including lack of a supportive peer group, of role models to follow, or of guidance in difficult situations, and risks in the immediate environment). Giese et al. (2003b) warn against using household form (e.g. nuclear family, grandmother caring for children, child-headed household) as a proxy for vulnerability.

In conclusion, it is relatively easy to come to a common definition of what we mean by a child or an orphan, after recognising that definition may vary between researchers and community members. But in determining whether a child is vulnerable (or negatively affected by HIV/AIDS), it is more difficult to set down a formal definition that can be used to easily identify research subjects. This is because there are many factors that can cause vulnerability in different combinations, and individual cases may need to be examined to determine degrees of vulnerability.

2.4   Should researchers focus on children orphaned by AIDS?

A major debate in the literature on the effects of the AIDS pandemic on children currently centres on whether children orphaned by AIDS (and other vulnerable children) are significantly worse off than other children. If so, should they be a special focus for research and interventions? In this section, we introduce the debate to set the backdrop for discussing issues of interest to stigma researchers in Chapter 3, and in Chapter 4 we will comment on some of the implications of this debate for policy-makers.

Orphans are a group that has historically been the focus of much western charity and concern. The family has been assumed to be of primary importance in socialisation, and in the absence of family support, society and the state have to undertake a certain responsibility for orphans. The AIDS pandemic will result in the illness and death of many young parents.

It is not surprising therefore that orphans have been the focus of much research and policy attention towards children affected by the AIDS pandemic. Orphans have been

---

2 H Meintjes, personal communication.

widely used as an index of the effects of the pandemic on children (Kamali et al. 1996; Lindblade et al. 2003). Illustrating the dire situation faced by orphans (and other vulnerable children) is helpful in justifying poverty-relief programmes (Consortium on Aids and International Development 2004; Gow & Desmond 2002). But some researchers argue that too much effort is being devoted to counting orphans, and too little effort to identifying broader risks to children's health and development (Subbarao & Coury 2003 in Richter et al. 2004).

2.4.1   Are orphans worse off than non-orphans?

It is important to assess whether there are specific problems faced by orphans, given the sheer numbers of children who will now lose one or more parents and the extent to which this will disrupt traditional family or community support structures for them. This is largely due to the AIDS pandemic: 'Since the HIV virus was first identified in 1981, more than three million children have been born HIV positive and the mothers of over 80 million children have died from AIDS' (UNAIDS 2000 in Amon 2002: 143). In eastern and southern African countries, household survey data in the late 1990s suggest that between 12 and 18 per cent of children aged between 7 and 14 were single or double orphans (Ainsworth & Filmer 2002).

In South Africa, the ASSA orphans model suggests that in the absence of medical or behavioural interventions:

> [t]he number of maternal orphans is expected to rise from roughly 990 000 in 2003 to 3.05 million in 2015, and the number of double orphans is expected to increase from 190 000 to two million by 2015. The total number of children under the age of 18 who have lost one or both parents is expected to peak at 5.6 million in 2014. (Cited in Meintjes et al. 2003: 27)

These numbers will hopefully be reduced with the introduction of prevention and treatment programmes.

There are a number of characteristics of the HIV/AIDS pandemic that have particularly negative material and psychosocial effects on children and their support systems. In the absence of widespread antiretroviral access, AIDS results in premature death of working age, sexually active adults, who are often parents. The cycle of poverty, child migration and food insecurity associated with adult deaths in households reduces the ability of families to care for children. Because AIDS orphans experience most of these serious effects of the pandemic, many researchers compare the circumstances of orphans (or AIDS orphans) to non-orphans as a proxy for measuring the impact of the pandemic on children.

A number of studies have found that orphans are less likely than non-orphans to have their basic material needs met, to have access to education, or to experience household stability (Makame et al. 2002; Muller et al. 1999;Ntozi & Mukiza-Gapere 1995). One study (Mturi & Nzimande 2003) found that although there were strong existing patterns of child labour in South Africa, the HIV/AIDS pandemic and associated poverty seems to have increased the trend towards children engaging in paid and unpaid labour. Younger children tend to suffer more from malnutrition and illness after being orphaned, while older orphans are more likely to be taken out of school (Nampanya-Serpell 1999). Other studies (discussed in Meintjes & Giese 2006), however, have found that orphans share problems with other poor children in terms of poverty, educational access

(Ainsworth & Filmer 2002; Case & Ardington 2004; Case et al. 2003; Kamali et al. 1996), care by adults (Urassa et al. 1997), and health outcomes (Crampin et al. 2005; Lindblade et al. 2003). Although orphans and children with chronically ill caregivers were poorer and had fewer indicators of good health, one study of about 2 000 children in Zambia and Rwanda (Chatterji et al. 2005) found no significant differences in school enrolment or age of sexual debut among orphans, children with chronically ill caregivers, and other children aged 6–19 years. Crampin et al. (2005) found that in their Malawian sample, children of HIV-positive mothers who survived, given their significantly higher mortality, did not experience significantly higher levels of stunting, being wasted, or reported ill-health compared to a control group.

The jury is still out therefore, on whether orphans are materially worse off than non-orphans. Or are the studies that do find significant differences simply badly designed? Meintjes and Giese (2006) argue that research studies on the material impact of the pandemic tend to target only orphans, AIDS orphans, or orphans and vulnerable children, they magnify small differences and generalise them beyond the study area, and link disadvantage to orphanhood without sufficient evidence. There is wide regional variation in the nature of the orphan problem (Abebe 2005), so national-level comparisons (Monasch & Boerma 2004) may not fully capture regional needs.

Some research in the psychosocial literature (both empirical and descriptive) has reported poor psychosocial functioning (mainly internalising problems)[3] in children orphaned by AIDS (Collins-Jones 1997; Lester et al. 2002). Other studies have found, however, that the psychosocial functioning of children orphaned by AIDS is not necessarily significantly poorer than that of other orphans, or indeed non-orphans (Cluver 2003; Wild et al. 2005). Negative effects of parental bereavement may be short-lived (Rotheram-Borus et al. 2005), and any negative effects, mainly internalising than externalising in nature, may in fact begin with parental illness and would not necessarily significantly increase with parental death (Forehand et al. 1998).

Are weak study designs to blame for the lack of agreement in psychosocial studies? Many of the psychosocial studies do not compare AIDS orphans with other orphans or children from the same community who are not orphaned (Wild et al. 2005). Children's ability to cope with adverse circumstances is affected by various mediating and moderating factors, which are often not controlled for.[4]

Wild et al. (2005) have identified the lack of a suitable control group as a key problem in studies that try to measure psychosocial impacts on individual children, debating whether children are fundamentally resilient or in need of psychosocial intervention when faced by parental death or illness. Wild et al. (2005) suggest that children orphaned by AIDS should be compared with other orphans and not with other children in general (Wild et al. 2005). Given the under-reporting of AIDS deaths (Grassly et al. 2004), control groups of other orphans should comprise children orphaned by accidents, murder and other non-health-related factors (Cluver, work in progress). Even so, Cluver notes that there are

---

3 The term 'internalising problems' has been used in the literature on children's responses to HIV/AIDS to describe psychosocial problems that are internalised by children (expressed through depression or withdrawal) rather than externalised (expressed through acting out behaviours). This is distinct from internalisation of stigma, discussed in the stigma literature, a term used to describe the process by which children or adults accept (or internalise) negative perceptions of them.

4 In Worsham et al.'s definition (1997: 204), moderating factors are factors that account for individual differences in children's responses to a stressor (e.g. age, severity of stressor), while mediating factors are those that account for the processes through which a stressor affects children's adjustment (e.g. coping methods).

issues (such as gang-related stigma, or post-traumatic stress disorder) that will have an impact on the psychosocial functioning of other orphans, quite apart from the stress of bereavement.

Since the AIDS pandemic will be responsible for creating vastly more orphans than existed in the past, and both orphanhood and HIV/AIDS contribute to the downward cycle of poverty in high prevalence areas, researchers on the material effects of the pandemic have not been as concerned about the lack of suitable control groups. Their research will, if anything, underestimate the material effects of the pandemic on children because many non-orphans will also suffer negative material effects.

In the absence of definitive evidence that orphans are significantly disadvantaged by being orphaned because of AIDS, do we need to improve our study designs to establish what is going on, or do we need to revisit the original problem in its entirety?

We wish to establish what the material and psychosocial effects of the AIDS pandemic are on children, with a view (in this paper, at least) to understanding the impact of stigma. One approach is to use rough proxies for the impact of AIDS, such as orphanhood, and to compare the situation of AIDS orphans to other orphans or to non-orphans. But, even if we could improve study designs by finding a suitable control group, it will not be easy to understand complex and wide-ranging effects of the HIV/AIDS pandemic such as stigma by comparing orphans with other children.

2.5   Why we need to stop focusing on orphans

Comparing orphans to non-orphans is, as a number of researchers have pointed out, not a good way of measuring the impact of the pandemic on children (Bray 2003; Meintjes & Giese 2006). Although increases in levels of orphanhood are due mainly to rising AIDS mortality (Meintjes et al. 2003), not all orphans are AIDS orphans. It is difficult to definitively identify AIDS orphans in the context of low disclosure rates. Also, not all AIDS-affected children are orphans.

The material and psychosocial impact of HIV/AIDS on children begins long before the death of the primary caregiver. Parental illness can be disruptive and distressing for children (Andiman 1995; Geballe et al. 1995; Giese et al. 2003b). In a situation of poverty, parental illness has severe financial implications for households, and children are often required to care for the ill parent, do housework and make money to survive. A national South African study found that although orphans were more likely to have dropped out of school than non-orphans, serious parental illness also adversely affected children's school attendance, increased school drop-out rates and decreased likelihood of immunisation (Brookes et al. 2004). Children are also affected by the illness and death of family members who are not caregivers (for example, siblings) and of caregivers or friends who may not be family members (Meintjes & Giese 2006).

The problems faced by orphans are not always due to orphanhood. In comparing orphans to non-orphans we have to control for other confounding factors: that orphans are more likely to be older and poorer than other children; that they are more likely to be in households with non-biological caregivers; and that parental death has psychosocial impacts on children independently of HIV/AIDS. There may in fact be some positive aspects to children's migration (increased access to schools, skills acquisition and better nutrition) (Henderson 2003 cited in Meintjes et al. 2003). The material, and possibly also the psychosocial, impact of orphanhood may also be tempered by the 'relatively smooth absorption' of orphans into existing fostering systems (Urassa et al. 1997). At some point, however, these systems become overloaded by the sheer number of orphans, and many countries in sub-Saharan African have already reached that point.

Finally, and perhaps most importantly, the problems faced by poor children orphaned by AIDS are often similar to those faced by other poor children in high-prevalence areas. In such areas, the problems experienced by children orphaned by AIDS 'reflect the effects of the multiple chronic adversities such as poverty, violence and single-parent households that often characterise the communities most affected by AIDS' (Wild et al. 2005). All poor children in regions with high HIV prevalence are 'likely to be affected by the ensuing deterioration of services, the weakening of social institutions and high levels of stress' (Richter 2004: 3; see also Giese et al. 2003b; Wild et al. 2005).

In poor, high-prevalence areas, the burden of HIV/AIDS spreads beyond households with HIV-positive members (Giese et al. 2003b). As fewer working-age adults are able to work, economies shrink, and households in general become poorer as more resources are spent on burying deceased relatives and caring for orphaned children. Five per cent of children under 14 in a national South African study provided care to non-household members with serious illness (Brookes et al. 2004).

Both orphans and non-orphans could routinely experience a sequence of different caregivers, frequent migrations, the lack of paternal figures, or separation from their biological siblings. A majority of children may now have to face illness and death of caregivers in the extended family system, whether or not they themselves actually become orphans before age 15 or 18. A large proportion of children in sub-Saharan communities where parents undertake migrant work have in the past been informally fostered with relatives, and have had to move to new communities and been separated from siblings and parents for extended periods (Bray 2003; Madhavan 2004).

2.6   Conclusion

In conclusion, researchers, development agencies and local communities often use different definitions of children, adolescents, orphans and vulnerable children. The same children may also fall into a number of different categories, and may move in and out of them.[5]

The key problem facing researchers is that it is difficult for study purposes to define a group of vulnerable children using easily and externally measurable characteristics of those children (e.g. orphanhood or poverty) as a proxy because so many factors interact in creating vulnerability in specific cases. This problem becomes particularly difficult when we also want to define a group of children as a control group to assess the impact of HIV/AIDS. These children have to be somehow less affected by HIV/AIDS in order to be part of the control group, even in a region of very high HIV prevalence, where they might be equally affected by problems such as poverty.

Specific issues, such as an inflated concern about orphans, have determined what data on children gets collected and how the data is interpreted. Comparing the experience of orphans and non-orphans has been used as a rough index of the material effects of the

---

5 H Meintjes, comments on this paper.

epidemic, but because even AIDS orphans are not the only children being affected by HIV/AIDS, defining study populations in this way will not be very helpful in identifying specific impacts of the pandemic, including the impact of HIV/AIDS-related stigma, on children.

Given the commonality of experience between orphans and many other children adversely affected by the AIDS pandemic, are there ways of defining study populations so that orphanhood is only one of the characteristics that could define vulnerability? Defining a group of children as 'orphans and vulnerable children' is an attempt to do this. There are two problems with using this approach to define study populations. First, the fact that vulnerability needs to be individually assessed makes it expensive to implement in a meaningful way. Second, the fact that defining what makes children vulnerable to disadvantage is rather dependent on what kind of vulnerability we want to measure. When we are trying to measure specific vulnerabilities, like disadvantages caused by HIV/AIDS-related stigma, our assessment of which children are likely to be affected might change.

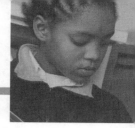

CHAPTER 3

The HIV/AIDS pandemic, stigma and children

Stigma is an important life concern for children infected and affected by HIV/AIDS (Brackis-Cott et al. 2003). Stigma can affect children directly when it leads to active discrimination, or status loss (which can exacerbate existing social marginalisation). It can also affect children indirectly when caregivers suffer the effects of stigma and discrimination, or when children or parents take certain courses of action (such as withdrawal) to avoid expected stigma or discrimination. HIV-negative children can be stigmatised by association with an HIV-positive caregiver (this is called courtesy stigma), and HIV-positive children may suffer direct stigma and discrimination as well as courtesy stigma.

In this section we describe and analyse current research on the HIV/AIDS pandemic, HIV/AIDS-related stigma and children. The literature on HIV/AIDS and children tends to focus on measuring the effects of the pandemic (including stigma) on children rather than on measuring stigmatising attitudes. Perhaps this is because children are perceived as innocent victims, or objects of discrimination in need of assistance (for other reasons for the focus on attitudes in adults see Deacon et al. 2005).

For the reasons discussed above, existing data comparing the material conditions or psychosocial adjustment of children orphaned by AIDS with other children (whether non-orphans or other orphans) cannot offer a detailed understanding of the impact of AIDS-related stigma on children. We can however develop some hypotheses from existing descriptive and quantitative studies on children on which future researchers can draw when designing their research. In this section we review existing literature to develop these hypotheses.

In this review we will focus on research that has theoretical, comparative or direct relevance to the sub-Saharan situation. The literature relating to children and HIV/AIDS stigma in regions with a type 1 epidemic, where predominant risk groups include gay men and drug users, is of variable applicability in high-prevalence, low-income regions with general, type 2 epidemics (for further explication of these types see Department of National Health and Population Development 1990 cited in Barrett et al. 1999).

African case studies are relatively well represented in research on the effects of the pandemic on children. This may be because the general nature of the pandemic in developing countries has highlighted the needs of poor families. However, African contexts differ from each other (Stein 2003a) and questions on stigma are limited or even absent from many surveys on effects of the pandemic on children.

3.1   Understanding the key research areas

There are large HIV/AIDS or health-related surveys such as the Demographic and Health Survey (DHS) that poll young people (usually over 15) on HIV knowledge, stigmatising attitudes and behaviours. The Horizons Program has developed a questionnaire on the well-being of AIDS-affected children, but results of this research could not be located by the authors. The Cape Area Panel Study (CAPS) study polls adolescents as well as adults on a range of issues including stigma. A national South African study run by the Human Sciences Research Council (HSRC) for the Nelson Mandela Foundation polled 15–24 year-olds on five stigma questions. There is also a WK Kellogg-funded HSRC project investigating the situation of orphans and vulnerable children in southern Africa (Davids et al. 2006; Gomo et al. 2006; Mahati et al. 2006; Simbayi et al. 2006).

In general, little of this data has been analysed specifically to understand youth attitudes and behaviours in comparison to adults (exceptions include Letamo 2004; Maugham-Brown in progress; Simbayi et al. 2006). An additional problem is that most studies on children are cross-sectional rather than longitudinal in design, which makes it difficult for researchers to disentangle the effects of orphanhood, poverty and factors like HIV/AIDS-related stigma in creating disadvantage for children. There are some longitudinal studies of children such as the South African Birth to Twenty study in which some questions on stigma have been asked,[6] but nothing has been published on this data currently.

There is a paucity of studies exploring children's attitudes towards people living with HIV/AIDS (exceptions include Castle 2004; Letamo 2004; and Lim et al. 1999). There has been some recent work on how adults stigmatise children affected by HIV/AIDS, and how this is related to stigmatisation of poverty, orphans and street children (Campbell et al. 2005; Foster et al. 1997; Foster & Williamson 2000; Hamra et al. 2005; Skinner et al. 2004).

Most KAB (Knowledge-Attitudes-Behaviours) research on children and HIV/AIDS focuses on prevention of high-risk behaviours rather than on stigma reduction (for example, Goodwin et al. 2004; Kaaya et al. 2002; Krasnik & Wangel 1990). Most of this kind of research thus tends to investigate adolescent knowledge and risk behaviours, especially substance abuse and unsafe sex, rather than children's attitudes towards people living with HIV/AIDS. In the same way, research on children and cancer in the 1980s (at a time when stigma about cancer was still quite high in the US) also focused on children's knowledge rather than their attitudes (Michielutte & Diseker 1982). Few of these quantitative studies explore children's experiences or expectations of stigma.

Stigma is usually discussed in the literature on psychosocial effects of the pandemic on children, which include the effects of stigma. Stigma associated with AIDS may isolate parents and children from family and community support, exacerbate their psychological distress and reduce access to education and healthcare. Increased material difficulties, some of which may be due to AIDS-related stigma, also have psychosocial consequences for children (discussed in Stein 2003a).

There is a growing amount of research on the psychosocial adjustment of children infected and affected by HIV/AIDS (Makame et al. 2002; Nagler et al. 1995; Stein 2003a; Wild 2001), and the problems parents face in the context of HIV/AIDS (Bond et al. 2000; Hough et al. 2003; Ingram & Hutchinson 1999; Lee & Rotheram-Borus 2002; Vallerand et al. 2005). While the KAB literature focuses on adolescents, the psychosocial literature focuses chiefly on orphans, mainly those under 15 (Grassly & Timaeus 2003). Most of the orphans studied are either not tested for HIV and, if not ill, assumed to be negative. There is a small but growing literature on the experiences of HIV-positive children, however, especially in wealthier countries (Gosling et al. 2004; Lewis 2001).

---

6 L Richter, personal communication.

Discrimination is generally addressed (albeit rather tangentially) in the more general literature on effects of the pandemic on children (Boler & Carroll 2003; Chase & Aggleton 2001; Daileader Ruland et al. 2005; Monasch & Boerma 2004). The literature on AIDS-related stigma and discrimination against children is aimed mainly at identifying examples of discrimination to direct advocacy for human rights work (Barrett et al. 1999; Clay et al. 2003; Strode & Barrett-Grant 2001). Documenting individual instances is useful in a legal sense but it does not tell us enough about the *extent* of discrimination experienced due to HIV/AIDS stigma.

A number of recent studies in Africa do draw on the experiences of children affected and infected by HIV/AIDS (Clacherty 2001; Clay et al. 2003; Giese et al. 2002; Giese et al. 2003b; Strode & Barrett-Grant 2001). Perhaps due to a general tendency to research children from an adult perspective, children's own experiences tend to be under-represented in the literature on children and HIV/AIDS. Most studies do not examine how children engage with stigmatising ideas at different stages of emotional and cognitive development (MacLeod & Austin 2003 are an exception).

Most of the research still represents children's experiences within the framework of measuring *effects* of the pandemic on children, predominantly by using standardised measures of psychosocial adjustment or poverty (Collins-Jones 1997; Laas 2004; Rotheram-Borus et al. 2005; Wild 2001). Once the key problems have been identified using these standardised measures, research on how stigma contributes to disadvantage requires more qualitative, process-sensitive studies exploring the *experiences* of children in greater detail (see for example Reyland et al. 2002).

The use of comparative work is particularly important given the paucity of research on children and AIDS-related stigma, and the potential existence of multiple stressors in a child's environment. In this literature review we therefore draw on the coping literature on children, which forms a useful theoretical framework for understanding the experience of stigma (Wolchik & Sandler 1997). We also refer to work on epilepsy and disability-related stigma (Carlton-Ford et al. 1997; Cramer et al. 1999; Green 2003; MacLeod & Austin 2003). Such stressors include:

- Family stressors, for example parental divorce (Emery & Forehand 1994 and Forehand et al. 1998b cited in Forehand et al. 1998; Lee 2001; Sandler et al. 1994; Wolchik & Sandler 1997) or poverty (Call et al. 2002);
- Chronic disease in the family, for example cancer (Compas et al. 1994 cited in Forehand et al. 1998; Michielutte & Diseker 1982; Pfeffer et al. 2000);
- Stigmatised illness or disability in children, for example obesity, epilepsy (Austin et al. 2004; Carlton-Ford et al. 1997; Devinsky et al. 1999; MacLeod & Austin 2003);
- Social prejudice, for example racism and sexism (Connolly 1998; Donald et al. 1995; van Ausdale & Feagin 2001).

Stein (2003a) makes the important point that comparative work on the psychosocial impact of poverty needs to be explored in understanding the relationship between material and psychosocial factors in assessing the impact of the AIDS pandemic on children:

> Those involved in the psychosocial support of children affected by AIDS need to acknowledge poverty, as well as the fact of orphanhood, as a primary psychological stressor. In addition, psychological support interventions cannot be effective without at the same time lessening the urgent material needs of OVCs. (2003a: 12)

We will now discuss how the literature on stigma, children and HIV/AIDS and the above comparative literatures inform the following hypotheses:

1. HIV/AIDS-related stigma exacerbates the negative effects of the pandemic on children and their support systems;
2. HIV/AIDS-related stigma towards children is framed within different social discourses;
3. Children stigmatise each other; and
4. Children experience HIV/AIDS-related stigma differently depending on their stage of emotional and cognitive development.

3.2 Hypothesis 1: HIV/AIDS-related stigma and discrimination exacerbates the negative effects of the pandemic on children

The few specific studies on children's experiences of stigma and discrimination (for example, Clay et al. 2003; Strode & Barrett-Grant 2001) have argued that children affected and infected by HIV/AIDS suffer considerable material and psychosocial disadvantage due to AIDS-related stigma both directly and indirectly (that is, through the effects of stigma and discrimination on caregivers). Strode and Barrett-Grant found that:

> Children whose parents are ill with AIDS or who have died of AIDS…report being marginalised and isolated from other children, being teased and gossiped about, being presumed to also be HIV-positive, and not receiving care. (2001: 16)

In examining the broader literature on the effects of the pandemic on children, however, it is less easy to identify specific effects of stigma. It is also difficult to separate the effects of stigma from the effects of parental death, poverty, orphanhood, and the provision of special services for children affected by HIV/AIDS or foster children. This is made more difficult by the fact that most research on the effects of the pandemic on children in high-prevalence areas uses a cross-sectional rather than a longitudinal design and does not ask detailed questions on stigma.

Given the compartmentalisation of the literature, but noting the importance of more integrated research on stigma in the future, we now explore the evidence for three sub-hypotheses, that stigma exacerbates the negative (a) psychosocial, (b) material and (c) indirect effects of the pandemic on children.

3.2.1 Hypothesis 1a: HIV/AIDS-related stigma exacerbates negative psychosocial effects of the pandemic on children

As the importance of understanding the psychosocial impact of the pandemic on children began to be realised, Geballe and Gruendel (1998) identified a number of 'unique challenges' faced by children in AIDS-affected households: disturbing clinical course of disease; uncertainty about when the infected person will die; multiple losses (including parental bereavement); (courtesy) stigma; family silence and secrecy; and additional multiple stressors (e.g. poverty). When speaking of HIV-positive children, one could also include direct stigmatisation and chronic illness on this list.

The specific combination of these challenges is what makes the effects of HIV/AIDS unique, because children in other contexts can of course experience poverty, bereavement, stigmatised illness and parental illness or death. Caregiver contraction of a chronic illness like AIDS can for example be disruptive and distressing for children. This can occur quite apart from stigmatisation, because the disease has a lengthy course. This requires adjustments to household functioning and resources as the sick adult requires hospitalisation or intensive home-based care, some of which may need to be done by the children themselves (Andiman 1995; Geballe & Gruendel 1998).

The extent of the stigmatisation associated with HIV/AIDS could distinguish the experiences of children in AIDS-affected households to some extent from those of children affected by less stigmatised diseases like cancer. But even children affected by relatively minor problems, and controllable, less life-threatening conditions like epilepsy like stuttering suffer greatly from stigma (Austin et al. 2004; Blood et al. 2003).

Stigma compounds the effects of other stressors (see Siegel & Gorey 1994; Gewirtz & Gossart-Walker 2000; Stein 2003a):

> The struggle to provide sustained, supportive relationships for their children is not unique to families with HIV disease. The effects of psychosocial deprivation, economic insufficiency, unemployment, parental drug abuse, and psychiatric impairment, as well as other chronic and fatal diseases can all impinge on these capacities. In AIDS-affected families, however, the issues are all the more powerful and problematic because they are compounded by the secrecy, stigma and certain fatality that are part of living with HIV infection. (Nagler et al. 1995: 72–73)

There does, for example, seem to be a link between stigma and increased depression. Epilepsy stigma research suggests a strong positive link between depression and epileptic adolescents' negative attitudes towards their own epileptic seizures (Dunn & Austin 1999). In children, negative attitudes about the parent's HIV-positive status (or their own) may be a predictor of depression (this may be somatised in the African context, see Cluver 2003).

Stigma is thought to hamper normal grieving processes, 'disenfranchising' children's grief. Silence around the cause of death can also hamper the grieving process.[7] Stigma can prevent children's acquisition of knowledge about HIV/AIDS, and it can delay or prevent parental disclosure to children or isolate children forced to keep the information secret (Letteney & Laporte 2004; Siegel & Gorey 1994; Vallerand et al. 2005).

For the purposes of this review the psychosocial literature will be divided broadly into three categories: research on psychosocial adjustment to bereavement; research on disclosure of HIV-status and other parenting issues; and research on special challenges faced by HIV-positive children. These will be discussed separately below.

3.2.1.1 Psychosocial adjustment to bereavement
Stigma is consequently one of the factors used to explain why children directly affected by HIV/AIDS (in this case, children orphaned by AIDS) suffer more psychosocial problems than other children:

> After controlling for the stressors mentioned in our study [going to bed hungry, not attending school, not receiving reward or praise], orphans still had significantly higher internalizing problem scores…[:] other unmeasured stressors [could include] lack of a caring adult to confide in, lack of other material resources, fear of being infected with HIV and *stigma associated with HIV infection*. (Makame et al. 2002: 464, our emphasis)

---

7 H Meintjes, comments on this paper.

Both descriptive and empirical studies have reported higher rates of psychosocial maladjustment in AIDS-affected children, especially orphans (Wild et al. 2005):

> Descriptive studies conducted in the USA have reported elevated levels of psychiatric problems including anxiety and depression among adolescents who had family members who were diagnosed with or had died of AIDS (Collins-Jones 1997; Lester, Rotheram-Borus & Lee, 2003; Pivnick and Villegas, 2000). One study (Hudis 1995) also reported high levels of acting-out behaviors in orphaned adolescents.

This kind of research has been criticised because it does not compare children's psychological state to that of control groups from the same community (Wild et al. 2005). But empirical studies with control groups (for example, Forehand et al. 1997; Forehand et al. 1998; Forehand et al. 1999) have also reported that children orphaned by AIDS experience more internalising problems than non-orphans.

Relatively few psychosocial studies on children affected by HIV/AIDS have been conducted in southern Africa (for reviews see Wild 2001; Stein 2003a). In a review of the psychosocial literature on Africa, Cluver (2005) found seven empirical studies that used a control group. All reported more internalising problems in children orphaned by AIDS than non-orphans (Atwine et al. 2005; Cluver & Gardner 2005; Makame et al. 2002; Poulter 1997; Sengendo & Nambi 1997; Wild et al. 2005). Forsyth et al. (1996, cited in Forsyth 2003) found that, compared to a control group from the same community, both caregiver and self-reported internalising symptoms were higher among children affected by HIV/AIDS, and significantly higher in children whose mothers showed symptoms of HIV/AIDS. Cluver (2003) found fewer differences than the other studies, finding only that children orphaned by AIDS were more likely to report having no good friend, somatic symptoms, and difficulty with concentration.

How do we find an appropriate control group? Hirsch (2001) and Wild et al. (2005) have suggested comparing children orphaned by AIDS to other orphans instead of only to non-orphans, because being orphaned creates psychosocial challenges for all children, not just HIV-affected ones.[8] It is also important to find ways of identifying representative groups of children who have been orphaned by AIDS[9] in contexts where children often do not know parental cause of death, and the opinions of other adults often have to be based on speculation given the necessity for healthcare workers to maintain confidentiality on patient records. Most current studies seem to rely on the reports of local NGOs or community members as to cause of death.

Based on adult research (Santana & Dancy 2000), we could expect that AIDS-related stigma would result in reduced self-esteem through internalisation in AIDS-affected children. But although Wild et al. (2005) comment on the significant stigma around HIV/AIDS in southern Africa, they found that other orphans reported lower self-esteem and higher depression and anxiety than either children orphaned by AIDS or non-orphans. Wild et al. (2005) thus suggest that 'while children orphaned as a result of AIDS do face some unique challenges, these additional stressors [including stigma, presumably] will have little effect on adolescents above and beyond the consequences of experiencing the

---

8 Factors associated with bereavement, such as inadequate parenting either before or after a parent's death, may be more harmful than bereavement itself: Harrington and Harrison (1999) suggest that childhood bereavement is not in itself a risk factor for mental or behavioural disorder.

9 H Meintjes, comments on this paper.

death of a parent and the loss of the love, support, guidance and security that parents ideally provide (Wild et al. 2005, citing Dane 1997)'.

In her study assessing the attachment security, anxiety, depression and conduct of children orphaned by HIV/AIDS compared with those orphaned by other causes, Hirsch (2001) found that children orphaned by AIDS fared no worse than other orphans on attachment security measures, and actually fared better on some measures. She concluded that 'when AIDS orphaned children receive the social services they require, they do not experience attachment disturbance, or subsequent behaviour problems' (Hirsch 2001: abstract).

Perhaps children orphaned by AIDS suffer fewer problems than other orphans because the former are more prepared for parental death. Some research in the US suggests that negative effects associated with HIV/AIDS-related stigma or parental bereavement may be counterbalanced by the protective effects of experiencing a long parental illness. Experiencing lengthy disruptions prior to the death of the parent may help children to adjust afterwards, and the long course of AIDS as an illness gives children time to adjust to the concept of a caregiver's impending death (Dane 1994; Dane & Levine 2005; Siegel & Gorey 1994; Siegel et al. 1996).

After a long illness the death of the parent may create a sense of closure and stability for children (Siegel & Gorey 1994; Dane 1994; Siegel et al. 1996). Using a sample of inner-city African American families, Forehand et al. (1999) found that there was no increase in psychosocial problems in a group of children after the mother's death. They suggest that the trauma of being orphaned may have been balanced out by the support experienced in the more stable households into which these children were adopted. In wealthier, more stable family environments in the US where the father was HIV-infected by blood transfusion (and not highly stigmatised) and the mother provided support, their children experienced no clinically elevated psychological problems compared to a control group (Forehand et al. 1997, 1998). However, these case studies may have greater applicability in the US, where parental drug use was frequently the cause of instability in the AIDS-affected families researched, and where child fostering of non-orphans is not widespread, even in poor families.

Extended illness does not necessarily result in better planning for the transition to an alternative caregiver. Siegel and Gorey (1994) make the point that fear of discussing death and the stigmatised nature of HIV/AIDS may make parents less likely to do custody planning for children in advance of their death. In their South African study, Giese et al. (2003b) found that few discussions were held with children about parental illness, death and custody planning. This was related to caregivers' reluctance to discuss death and illness with minors, and to fears of stigma and discrimination if they cannot keep the information secret.

Whatever the merits of these arguments, there are some more fundamental problems with using the psychosocial data to understand the impact of AIDS-related stigma on children. The Hirsch study did not include a control group of non-orphans and had a small sample size (16 children in one group and 18 in the other). Wild et al. (2005) have noted some problems with their sampling. Perhaps more importantly, neither study effectively separates AIDS-affected children from less-affected or non-affected children. Some AIDS-related parental deaths may be included in the 'other orphan' category because of ignorance or misreporting of cause of death. Non-orphaned children may suffer courtesy stigma directed at their HIV-positive parents, siblings or other caregivers. HIV-positive children who are not orphaned may suffer direct stigma and discrimination. There was no specific stigma data collected so it is difficult to assess in what way stigma might have affected the psychosocial status of the children.

If this is the case, the above data may be telling us very little about AIDS-related stigma at all. The jury is still out on whether HIV/AIDS-related stigma has a significant effect on the psychological functioning of children orphaned by HIV/AIDS. Nevertheless, the psychological research raises important questions about the nature and impact of AIDS-related stigma on children. Are the psychosocial effects of AIDS-related stigma spread evenly throughout the population of AIDS-affected children, including children orphaned by AIDS, HIV-positive children and children with HIV-positive household members, making it difficult to pick them up in the empirical data discussed above? Are these effects less significant than expected? Or are they easily mitigated by providing support to children? Is measuring psychosocial adjustment a good index of the effects of stigma and discrimination on children?

3.2.1.2 Mediating and mitigating factors

As a number of researchers have pointed out, it is difficult to interpret the results of studies comparing the psychosocial adjustment of different categories of children unless we take account of mediating and mitigating factors. The psychosocial impact of caregiver illness and death may be mediated and moderated by the continuity and stability of the living environment, the quality of external social support, the severity of parental illness, the degree of parental depression, the age of the child, characteristics of the child (e.g. coping strategies), and so on (Wild 2001; Wild et al. 2005; Wolchik & Sandler 1997). Since the methods of coping with parental illness and bereavement are affected by the age of the child, and children orphaned by AIDS may not have the same age profile as non-orphans or other orphans (Case & Ardington 2004), it is advisable to control for age.

The psychosocial impact on children of the illness and death of a parent depends to a large extent on what other support structures can be put in place. The type of support may also influence the way children experience and cope with stigma. As Wild et al. (2005) point out, NGO support for the children orphaned by AIDS in their sample could have encouraged these children to adopt better coping strategies to deal with bereavement and any AIDS-related stigma.

As Bray (2003) and others have noted, it is important to be sensitive to the fluid and often non-nuclear nature of living arrangements in determining mediating or mitigating factors. A child's living arrangements prior to parental death are a significant factor in determining the psychosocial impact of parental bereavement.[10] For example, if the child has never met the biological father, the mother has been working at a distance for some time, and the child is being cared for by the grandmother, parental illness and bereavement will have less impact than if the mother or father were living with the child at the time, and it may have fewer psychosocial impacts on the child than the death of the grandmother.

The nature and extent of disclosure of the illness, and reactions to disclosure will also affect how children cope with caregiver illness and death, or their own illness. Some researchers have developed the notion of a 'stigma trajectory' showing how people living with HIV/AIDS have to deal with different levels of stigma as they show more signs of

---

10 L Cluver, comments on this paper.

illness (Alonzo & Reynolds 1995). It is thus important to develop measures of disclosure, consequences of disclosure and stage of illness in studies that try and assess the impact of stigma on children affected by HIV/AIDS.

3.2.1.3 Disclosure, parenting and HIV

From a public health point of view, disclosure of HIV status is seen as beneficial in encouraging PLWHA to access services, improve treatment compliance, and, in the case of parental HIV, to engage in custody planning and bereavement preparation for their children. Disclosure reduces the need for secrecy and can also reduce stigma around HIV/AIDS if it normalises the disease (Paxton 2002). Secrecy and silence about illness and death have been identified as problematic for children in particular because in the absence of a frank discussion and opportunities to ask questions, children may have very disturbing and frightening thoughts on these subjects (Daniel 2005; Nagler et al. 1995). Disclosure is a process that needs to be structured to accommodate parental capacity to cope with making the disclosure in a supportive way and the child's capacity to receive it.

There is a reasonably comprehensive body of research, at least for developed countries, in the psychosocial literature on disclosure, parenting and HIV (Flanagan-Klygis et al. 2002; Lee & Rotheram-Borus 2002; Lester et al. 2002; Lipson 1994; Nehring et al. 2000; Schonfeld 1997; Vallerand et al. 2005; Wiener et al. 1996; Wiener et al. 2000). For a review of this literature see Stein (2003a), who notes the paucity of African work on disclosure.

Lee and Rotheram-Borus suggest that the process of disclosing parental HIV status to children is similar to disclosure of other sensitive information and disclosure to adult sexual partners (Lee & Rotheram-Borus 2002). Clearly, disclosure of HIV status within families could be comparable to disclosure of other serious illnesses or issues like drug abuse. In research on childhood cancer, it has been suggested that parents tend to act as information executives, managing information about the illness to try and protect children. Full disclosure of medical information (or the consequences of illness) is not easy for parents who wish to appear optimistic and in control, nor is it always desired by children (Young et al. 2003).

Children often know more than they are being told. In a study on disclosure about childhood cancer, Claflin and Barbarin (1991) found that parents told younger children less about their illness than older children to spare them from being overwhelmed. However, children of different ages in this study reported similar levels of distress, suggesting that 'nondisclosure fails to mask the salient and distressing aspects of the disease' (Claflin & Barbarin 1991: 169). Children of drug users also tend to have a detailed awareness of their parents' drug problem, even if the parents impose the fiction that drugs are not a problem in the family. Silencing the discussion about drug dependence at home simply inhibits children from unburdening to others (Barnard & Barlow 2003).

The literature on disclosure, and that on discrimination, provide the most compelling evidence that HIV/AIDS-related stigma is a critical problem for children affected by HIV/AIDS in a stigmatising society. There are two main areas of investigation in the literature: disclosure of parental HIV-positive status to children and the disclosure of children's HIV-positive status to families and others. The findings on stigma in these areas of investigation will now be discussed in turn.

3.2.1.4 Disclosing parental HIV status to children

Some people rationally choose not to disclose their status because they anticipate little support or fear negative consequences of disclosure (Stein 1996). In South Africa, adult disclosure rates in general are low (Pawinski & Lalloo 2001). Women in a sexual partnership who test first through antenatal services and then disclose their status to their partner are often blamed for infecting the partner. Because the mother is highlighted as the recipient of treatment in prevention of mother-to-child transmission programmes, HIV-positive mothers are also often blamed for infecting their children (Policy Project et al. 2003).

Stigma and discrimination, and expectations of stigma, seem to affect parental decision-making on disclosure processes. Lewis (2001) suggests that non-disclosure of HIV status to children is rooted in the stigma associated with AIDS, rather than its nature as a terminal or chronic illness. Higher expected stigma reduces the likelihood of adult PLWHA disclosing to significant others (Clark et al. 2003; Mawn 1999; Petrak et al. 2001 and Pierret 2000 cited in Lee & Rotheram-Borus 2002). In Khayelitsha, Cape Town, the AIDS and Society Research Unit of the University of Cape Town found that HIV-positive women delayed disclosure to their children of their HIV status because of high expectations of stigma (Stein 2003a). However, Ostrom et al. (2006) have suggested several problems with current research on the interaction between expected or perceived stigma and parental disclosure. Most of this research is not empirical, or does not use scales adapted for measuring expected stigma, making it difficult to compare levels of expected stigma between respondents. Also, most studies do not distinguish between disclosure to all children and disclosure to some children in analysing disclosure patterns (Ostrom et al. 2006).

Parental expectations of stigma can delay but do not prevent disclosure of parental status (Lee & Rotheram-Borus 2002). US studies found that disclosure decisions taken by HIV-positive parents usually depend on the developmental stage of the child and the degree of parental illness (Vallerand et al. 2005). The main trigger for disclosure in these studies seems to be preparing children for parental illness and death. HIV-positive parents were more likely to disclose to their children when the parents were sicker and when they had known of their HIV status for longer (Lee & Rotheram-Borus 2002). Parents try and prepare children reasonably well in advance: about half the parental disclosures occurred two to four years prior to parental death, while only seven per cent occurred within the last year before death.

African case studies on disclosure suggest a slightly different pattern of parental disclosure. African mores (see Williamson 2000 in Stein 2003a) that proscribe death-related discussions, especially with children, in some cases reduced the likelihood of disclosure about the nature of parental illness, even after parental death (Marcus 1999 in Stein 2003a). Daniel (2005) found that in Botswana, children aged under 14 are still generally excluded from funerals and discussions about death. Bereavement planning concerns remain important, however. In a Ugandan study, (Gilborn et al. 2001) found that most of the older orphans who knew a parent who had died of AIDS were in favour of parental disclosure. Being able to plan for the future was one of three main reasons both children and parents in that study were in favour of parental disclosure, although only 57 per cent of the HIV-positive parents had actually disclosed to their children.

Is parental disclosure good for children? Stein (2003a) argues that disclosure prior to parental death allows children to come to terms with impending bereavement, say goodbye to their parent, and preserve and foster a relationship of trust and openness between parent and child. In two US studies, knowledge of parental HIV status actually reduced anxiety levels and allowed children to prepare for parental death (Rosenheim et al. 1985 and West et al. 1991 in Forsyth 2003).

However, parental disclosure of HIV status can be associated with long-lasting negative consequences for both parents and children, including more problem behaviours in adolescents, negative family events and greater stigma and discrimination (Lee & Rotheram-Borus 2002). This negative finding may be partly due to the relationship between the timing of parental disclosure and stressful live events such as resumption of drug use in their sample.

One of the negative results of parental disclosure to children may be the burden of keeping the disclosure secret – if parents are concerned that children will tell others, thus increasing stigma and discrimination towards them or the family in general. A recent study (Murphy et al. 2002) suggested that children find it stressful to keep the secret of parental HIV status. Nevertheless, children seemed highly motivated to keep their parent's status secret and in that study only shared the information inappropriately in less than 10 per cent of cases. This is consistent with low rates of disclosure of sensitive issues by children in other contexts (see below).

Whether or not parents have disclosed to their children may not be the critical factor in whether children cope with parental illness. Other possible influences on child coping may include the current health status of the parent and the amount of responsibility for parental or familial problems the child bears as a result of this. Reviewing a number of studies on parental HIV, Forsyth (2003) suggests that the parent's health status (that is, whether they are symptomatic or not) is a greater determinant of the mental health of the child than whether the child has been informed of the diagnosis. When parents are obviously sick, children will worry anyway. They may know something is wrong, even where they do not know the exact details.

Responsibility for parental care may increase as parental health status declines, but it may also increase when parents disclose more about their problems, which is sometimes framed by parents, or interpreted by children, as a sharing of responsibility. Research into children's coping in divorced families has suggested that girls may worry more about their mother's problems after the problems have been discussed with them. Disclosure of problems experienced by mothers after divorce to their daughters was associated with increased psychological distress in the daughters (Koerner et al. 2002). Other studies suggest that adolescent girls with sick mothers tend to be given more responsibilities and receive more maternal confidences, which partly explains why they experience greater distress than other children in a family (Worsham et al. in Wolchik & Sandler 1997).

In conclusion, the literature on parental disclosure suggests that expectations of stigma and discrimination as a result of disclosure may delay but not prevent parents from disclosing their HIV-positive status to their children, especially once they become ill. Nevertheless, children of HIV-positive parents may know that something is wrong before disclosure occurs. After public parental disclosure, children may experience increased stigma and discrimination from others. If others do not know, children have to bear the pressure of keeping the secret.

3.2.1.5 Disclosure of children's HIV status

There are slightly different issues involved in disclosing children's HIV-positive status, for parents and the children, but stigma and discrimination also play an important role in determining the process and effects of disclosure.

Parents very frequently justify not telling children (especially younger children) of their (the children's) own HIV-positive status because of expected stigma and discrimination should the children in turn disclose to others (Lester et al. 2002). Giese et al. reported in their South African study that:

> [A] non-symptomatic HIV-positive caregiver said that she would definitely not tell any of the neighbours about her child's suspected HIV-positive status because 'people might not want to touch her and when she is older they might stop their children from interacting with her and maybe all of us as a family might be stigmatised'. (2003a: 69)

Even when children do know their status, various studies have pointed to children's reluctance to disclose their HIV status to their peers. This suggests high levels of expected peer stigmatisation around HIV. The nature and effects of peer stigmatisation by children will be discussed more fully in the next section. Low rates of child disclosure due to fear of peer stigmatisation can be found among adolescents with epilepsy (Austin et al. 2004) and those who stutter (Blood et al. 2003).

The timing and nature of disclosure cannot always be controlled. HIV-positive children may experience direct stigma and discrimination because of secondary disclosure,[11] when others interpret physical signs of their illness or the treatment thereof as evidence that they have HIV/AIDS. Frequent illness may be interpreted as a sign of HIV/AIDS by other children and by adults. Stigma associated with the stunting of growth caused by HIV infection has psychological consequences for HIV-positive children in wealthy countries where other children are unlikely to be stunted through malnutrition (Forsyth 2003). Anxiety about physical differences due to stunting is a serious problem for HIV-positive children in South Africa[12] and in Cote de Ivoire (Dago-Akribi & Cacou Adjoua 2004). Children who take antiretroviral medication may experience physical and cognitive side-effects from the medication, and they may find that taking pills results in secondary disclosure.

Although Rosenheim and Reicher (1985 in Forsyth 2003) suggest that disclosure to children about parental terminal illness may reduce anxiety in the children, knowing one's own status may not always be a good experience for children. In one large US study, HIV-positive children who knew their diagnosis experienced a significantly elevated incidence of psychiatric hospitalisation compared to children who did not know they were HIV-positive and to children who were HIV-negative. The children were mainly hospitalised for depression, behavioural disorders and thoughts of suicide disorders, which were psychosocial rather than medical in origin (Gaughan et al. 2004).

It could be that the Gaughan sample was skewed because symptomatic cases may have been more likely to know their HIV status and/or caregivers may have been more likely to hospitalise children who knew their status – having symptoms, rather than knowing one's HIV status, may be what depresses children most. But Gaughan et al. (2004) found

---

11 We have defined secondary disclosure as disclosure through other means than telling someone you are HIV-positive or have AIDS.
12 R Nassen, personal communication.

that CD4 count and viral load (which measure disease status and are a proxy for level of associated infections) were not significantly associated with first hospitalisations. So it seems that for children, simply knowing one's HIV-positive status may actually increase the risk of experiencing psychiatric problems.

In conclusion, whereas the literature on psychosocial adjustment does not unambiguously demonstrate that stigma is a problem for children affected by HIV/AIDS, the literature on disclosure is very clear on this subject. Stigma, discrimination and expected stigma and discrimination play a major role in influencing parental and children's decision-making on, and the impact of, disclosure of HIV-status. Low rates of disclosure impede children's access to support and services. In this light, it is important for more research on disclosure to be done with children in the African context.

3.2.1.6 Psychosocial research on HIV-positive children

Adolescents and younger children can contract HIV perinatally, through breast feeding, through contaminated needles (unsterilised hospital equipment or drug use), through transfusions, and through penetrative sex, including rape. High rates of maternal infection, child rape, drug abuse and early sexual debut in Southern Africa contribute to a relatively high incidence of HIV among youth (Newell et al. 2004).

Yet most psychosocial research has focused on HIV-negative children of HIV-positive parents. Researchers have wanted to isolate the effects of AIDS-related orphanhood on children from the effects of actually having HIV. The main concern of intervention agencies has been to reach children who have a chance of surviving to adulthood, which until recently was confined to HIV-negative children. With increasing access to antiretroviral therapy for children, this is beginning to change. An index of this change is a growing body of papers on medical care for HIV-positive children (for example, Goulder et al. 2001; Granados et al. 2003; Khongkunthian et al. 2001) and public health services for them (Jeena et al. 2005; Lyon & Woodward 2003).

In the context of poor antiretroviral access, low rates of testing and low disclosure rates it is presumably also difficult to find a large and representative group of HIV-positive children to survey about stigma except as part of larger household surveys that test for HIV. Recent studies suggest that about 5 per cent of South African children (2–18 years) are infected by HIV, a prevalence figure that remains fairly constant across the age groups. Children of African descent, in poor households, and those living in informal settlements are more likely than other children to be HIV-positive (Brookes et al. 2004). This South African pattern of age-related prevalence in children is more uniform than that found in the household survey in Chimanimani district in Zimbabwe where about three per cent of the children aged 2–14 were HIV-positive, but 5.3 per cent of 15–18 year-olds were HIV positive (Gomo et al. 2006).

HIV-positive children are of particular interest to stigma research because they may experience more intense and direct effects of stigma and discrimination than HIV-negative children of HIV-positive parents. A minority of the psychosocial studies look specifically at HIV-positive children, however (exceptions include Forsyth 2003; Gaughan et al. 2004; Gosling et al. 2004; Kmita et al. 2002; Krener & Miller 1989; Lewis 2001; Melvin et al. 2005). Research that addresses stigma and focuses on HIV-positive youth in Africa is minimal (Dago-Akribi & Cacou Adjoua 2004), but some more general studies have referred to HIV-positive children's experiences of stigma and discrimination (Strode & Barrett-Grant 2001).

Comparing the psychosocial adjustment of children infected by HIV to other children can be useful in assessing the impact of stigma on psychosocial adjustment, but there may be a number of confounding factors. Chronic disease may affect psychosocial adjustment independently of stigma. Nelms (1989) found that children with less life-threatening and less stigmatised chronic diseases like asthma and diabetes suffered significantly higher levels of depression than well children. There are also medical triggers for depression in people with HIV/AIDS (Valente 2003).

At later stages of AIDS, children may develop developmental and cognitive difficulties associated with the effect of the virus on brain function (Gosling et al. 2004; Forsyth 2003). AIDS dementia complex is untreatable (Krener & Miller 1989; Weisberg & Ross 1989) and in the absence of effective treatments, may delay development and lead to HIV-positive children being progressively less able than other children to develop coping strategies around stigma, and to assess the risks and benefits of disclosure or withdrawal in specific situations because of their illness.

3.2.1.7 Conclusion: psychosocial effects on children

Psychometric research is a necessary tool for investigating AIDS-related stigma and children, but careful consideration should be given to choosing appropriate study designs. In most of the psychosocial studies, stigma tends to be treated as a self-evident explanation for differences that cannot be explained by other factors, rather than as an object of inquiry. It is difficult to measure the extent of stigma and its effects, and especially difficult to measure this in children. But with some notable exceptions, few studies actually try to do this.

For the purposes of researching stigma, existing empirical studies on the psychosocial effects of bereavement fail to distinguish sufficiently between children who might be affected by HIV/AIDS stigma and those who are less affected or unaffected. Indeed, it is difficult to find a group of children who are not affected by AIDS in high HIV-prevalence areas. To identify suitable control groups we need to develop a complex range of criteria, eliciting information that is not always fully known or understood by children, or volunteered to researchers.

It seems clear, however, that simply identifying internalising or externalising problems is too blunt a measure of children's experiences of stigma and its effects on them. We need more research on disclosure and on the experiences of HIV-positive children. We also need to ask more questions about stigma in both cross-sectional and longitudinal studies.

3.2.2 Hypothesis 1b: stigma exacerbates negative material effects of the pandemic on children

The AIDS pandemic has had serious negative material effects on children in developing countries, increasing poverty, malnutrition, and orphanhood and reducing access to services (Davids et al. 2006; Giese et al. 2003b; Monasch & Boerma 2004; Richter et al. 2004). When children in South Africa affected by AIDS (mainly orphans) were asked to name and rank their key problems (Giese et al. 2003b), they focused on the lack of food, shelter, clothes, school fees and equipment. Gossip and mistreatment from schoolmates, family and neighbours were also mentioned.

Studies on AIDS, children and stigma (for example, Strode & Barrett-Grant 2001) argue that stigma and discrimination exacerbate the negative material effects of the pandemic on children. However, the lack of systematic inquiry into the extent of the problem means that we often do not know how much stigma and related discrimination negatively affects children, or to what extent material disadvantages experienced by AIDS-affected children are exacerbated by AIDS-related stigma. Equally, where material disadvantage is not present, or not obvious (given the questions we have asked and the way we have cut the data cake), we tend to assume that stigma is not a problem.

In a study of mortality and physical well-being in orphans in Malawi, for example, researchers found that, although children of HIV-positive mothers suffered significantly higher mortality, compared to a control group, 'neither maternal HIV status nor orphanhood was associated with stunting, being wasted, or reported ill-health' in those who survived. The authors suggest therefore that 'the extended family in this society has not discriminated against surviving children whose parents have been ill or have died as a result of HIV/AIDS' (Crampin et al. 2005: 389). This may well be the case, but in the absence of specific inquiry into stigma and discrimination we cannot say for sure.

We will now examine some of the evidence that AIDS-related stigma and discrimination do exacerbate the material effects of the pandemic on children. The type, extent and effects of stigma may differ depending on situational context: school, healthcare setting, community and home. Work addressing each context will therefore be examined separately.

3.2.2.1 Households

Strode and Barrett-Grant (2001) found evidence of stigma and discrimination against children affected by HIV/AIDS in South African households, including provision of separate eating utensils, isolation from other members of the household, greater expectations of work contributions, and lack of care, emotional support and attention. In a Zambian study, fostered children whose parents died of HIV/AIDS described experiences of different forms of mistreatment or abuse in the household, including being given a heavier workload than other children at home; needing to 'work for their keep'; sexual abuse; and receiving harsher punishments (Clay et al. 2003: 24). These children also experienced withholding of food, education or shelter (Clay et al. 2003). Some orphaned children reported similar abuse in a Zimbabwean study, although loss of inheritance does not seem widespread (Mahati et al. 2006).

The situation of growing poverty affecting households in many of these countries makes it harder for households to absorb additional non-productive members. Both desperately poor parents and some guardians were reported in Zimbabwe to be either encouraging, or turning a blind eye to, prostitution by children in their care (Mahati et al. 2006). Newly arrived, non-biological children in a household may be required to work harder than the biological children of caregivers as a matter of course, but a significant proportion of other stigma and discrimination reported in the studies above seems to be related to fear of infection from HIV and to moral judgement (symbolic stigma). Refusal of home-based care services or family assistance because of fear of stigma surrounding disclosure of HIV status may increase the burden on children caring for symptomatic HIV-positive parents (Baggaley et al. 1999).

Children do face stigma and discrimination from local communities in general. As this will be more fully discussed in the section on the content of stigma (hypothesis 2) issues around the relationship between poverty and (resource-based) stigma will be addressed there.

In conclusion, much of the research suggests that children affected by HIV/AIDS who are formally or informally fostered in other households may be stigmatised and discriminated against. This may be because such children are perceived as a financial burden to the new household, because they are perceived as outsiders or newcomers, or because of HIV/AIDS-related stigma. Further research needs to be done to determine which factors are most important in driving this phenomenon, and how they can be addressed in a situation of increasing poverty and child migration. This kind of discrimination, aimed at the least powerful members of a household, and enacted within that household, is probably the most widespread, the most easily hidden and the most difficult to address.

3.2.2.2 Education

Stigma affects children's access to education. Some HIV-positive children are actively excluded from schools. In South Africa, the National Policy on HIV/AIDS for Learners and Educators now prohibits unfair discrimination against learners and educators in schools, but enforcement of such policies is generally weak and many children still complain of ostracism at school (Strode & Barrett-Grant 2001).

Chase and Aggleton (2001) reported from Zambia that children whose parents had died as a result of HIV/AIDS were sometimes taunted by other children and were thus reluctant to go to school. Caregivers reported feeling it was unsafe to send children who are HIV-positive to school for fear of discrimination and bullying. A Zimbabwean study reported instances of verbal abuse and blaming towards OVC in schools (Mahati et al. 2006). In Mozambique, a recent study reported stigma and discrimination at school as reducing school attendance among a small proportion of OVC (Save the Children Alliance & Hope for African Children Initiative 2004). Similar reports came from a Scottish study with HIV-negative children of HIV-positive parents reporting reluctance to disclose to schoolmates for fear of being discriminated against, or treated differently (Cree et al. 2004). Some participants were supported by friends on disclosure, but others were silenced by fear and some were actively 'slagged' at school by friends and classmates in a range of friendly and unfriendly ways.

HIV/AIDS-related stigma clearly affects children's school experiences. To what extent can lower attendance at school by AIDS-affected children be explained by other factors like maternal death, a child's gender, bereavement trauma, or poverty, however? A Ugandan study found that a far lower proportion of HIV-positive children of school-going age attended school compared to other children, explained in the study by ill-health or lack of school fees (O'Hare et al. 2005).

Using data on children in sub-Saharan Africa from 19 Demographic and Health surveys, conducted in 10 countries between 1992 and 2000, one study found that while orphans generally lived in poorer households, this was not why they experienced educational disadvantage:

> Children living in households headed by non-parental relatives fare systematically worse than those living with parental heads, and those living in households headed by non-relatives fare worse still. Much of the gap between the schooling of orphans and non-orphans is explained by the greater tendency of orphans to live with more distant relatives or unrelated caregivers. (Case et al.: 2)

In a longitudinal study in South Africa, Case and Ardington (2004) found that in the same household in KZN, an orphan's education would be allocated fewer resources than non-orphans. The death of a mother, specifically, creates significant disadvantage for children. Maternal death is the main predictor of lower educational status for orphans.

> Maternal and double orphans are at significant disadvantage with respect to their schooling, with or without controls for household characteristics. Specifically, children who have lost mothers have fallen more than a third of a year behind other children in school, on average. They are 3 percentage points less likely to be enrolled in school and, controlling for household socioeconomic status, children who have lost mothers have less spent on their education-related expenses, relative to other children on average. (Case & Ardington 2004: 15)

The study showed that maternal death adversely affects the education status of children independently of poverty, the child's health status, the child's gender, or death of the father, either because mothers are education champions and/or because the child is traumatised by the death of the mother.

Longitudinal data from studies like Case and Ardington (2004), and data from a large multi-country study Case et al. (2002) suggest that poverty and the gender of the child play less of a role in determining educational disadvantage for orphans than we might have expected.[13] The biological relationship between caregiver and orphan, and the gender of the deceased biological parent, seem to have a much more significant impact on how they are treated. This kind of study highlights the importance of understanding the precise interaction between factors that cause disadvantage in schooling.

Maternal and paternal bereavement thus has a differential impact on children. Mothers and fathers generally perform different family roles in relation to children (e.g. mothers generally do more emotional care-work and fathers tend to provide more material support). Fathers' contributions are more likely to be lost through migration or desertion, violent death in the case of younger fathers, and HIV/AIDS in the case of older fathers. Mothers' contributions are more likely to be lost through HIV/AIDS, which is more likely to affect younger mothers.[14]

The role of HIV/AIDS-related stigma in this process not clear, since neither HIV nor stigma data were collected in the longitudinal studies cited above. It could be hypothesised that AIDS-related stigma towards children is stronger on the death of a mother than a father, which may be one additional reason why a mother's death results in greater educational disadvantage than the death of a father in regions of high HIV-prevalence. It is likely, given the discussion on 'mother-cussing' (see Hypothesis 4), that children would face greater stigma and likelihood of disclosure in regard to their mother's HIV status than to the status of their father, especially in the context of high adult male migrancy and abandonment by fathers.

If children also face greater stigmatisation from peers than from other adults, or experience more regular and more serious stigma and discrimination at school than in other contexts, schooling experiences could easily be affected negatively by AIDS-related stigma.

---

13 These findings may not be generalisable. Using the broader South African October Household Survey data, Ainsworth and Filmer (2002), found that maternal orphans had higher enrolment rates than both paternal orphans and non-orphans. Thanks to H. Meintjes for making this point.
14 D Skinner, personal communication.

In conclusion, although there are a few cases of active exclusion from schools, this is becoming less common and easier to challenge. However, stigma can negatively affect children's experiences of school and may also be a contributory factor in reducing school attendance, especially where children have lost their mothers to HIV/AIDS.

3.2.2.3 Healthcare

Stigma affects children's access to healthcare facilities. Among African-American adolescents in San Francisco, especially women, expectations of stigma by health care workers were a significant barrier to seeking health care (Cunningham et al. 2002). Adolescent adherence to treatment regimes is also strongly associated with fear of social stigma (Pugatch et al. 2002). It is not clear whether younger HIV-positive children, who may well be perceived by nurses as less blameworthy than adolescents, would have the same fear of healthcare services.

In an environment of general scarcity and low treatment availability, investing time and money in caring for an HIV-positive child may seem like a waste of resources to parents, caregivers and healthcare workers (International HIV/AIDS Alliance 2003). In a Ugandan study, HIV-positive children did not return to the clinic for follow-up treatment because of stretched resources in vulnerable families (O'Hare et al. 2005).

Caregivers who are afraid of stigmatisation or discrimination towards themselves or the children may hesitate to disclose the status of HIV-positive children by taking them for treatment (Strode & Barrett-Grant 2001). In a South African study, researchers found that only five of the 40 mothers actually returned with their child to the Red Cross Children's hospital for follow-up visits after diagnosis – reasons given were to avoid being stigmatised, or because they were asymptomatic, because clinic visits cost money, and because post-test counselling was poor (Robertson & Ensink 1992).

One recent study (Tanzania Stigma-Indicators Field Test Group 2005) found that fewer Tanzanian healthcare workers report holding stigmatising attitudes towards PLWHA (one-fifth to one-third of respondents) than observe discriminatory behaviour towards PLWHA, such as the taking of unnecessary precautions, enforced testing or unauthorised disclosure (about 60 per cent of respondents). Giese et al. (2003b), in a South African study specifically on children, found that children were often referred to tertiary healthcare facilities for HIV testing and treatment because clinic staff felt they lacked the capacity to do so. There may be medical issues that a small clinic cannot address, but unnecessary referral of HIV-positive patients was also reported by 15 per cent of respondents in the Tanzanian study.

The Tanzanian work and Giese et al. (2003b) found little evidence of healthcare workers refusing to treat HIV-positive people (or children), although the quality of care for HIV-positive people was sometimes lower. It is possible, however, that refusal of care may be under-reported by healthcare providers. In the Save the Children study (Strode & Barrett-Grant 2001), an NGO called Thandanani that cares for HIV-positive children, the Children's Rights Centre in Kwa-Zulu Natal, South Africa, and children living with HIV/AIDS all reported cases of healthcare workers refusing care, or providing inferior care, to children who were HIV positive because of their HIV status, making them feel ashamed of their status.

In conclusion, children's access to healthcare could be affected by HIV/AIDS stigma in various ways. Adolescents are particularly vulnerable to fears of social stigma, and may be reluctant to expose themselves to moral judgements by nursing staff on their sexual activity. Children's caregivers may be reluctant to disclose their status or the children's status by bringing them to clinics or hospitals. They may also be reluctant, in a situation of increasing poverty, to spend the money on transporting children who are not their own, and/or who are expected to die soon. Healthcare workers could refuse care, or provide lower standards of care in both direct and indirect ways (e.g. by unnecessary referrals). The paucity of treatment education around HIV-positive children and the reduced availability of treatment suitable for children may be a broader, underlying issue in the healthcare system.

3.2.2.4 Conclusions: Material effects of HIV/AIDS-related stigma on children

Although there is some evidence that HIV/AIDS-related stigma has material negative effects on children's treatment and care in the household, in healthcare settings and at school, it is difficult to assess from the descriptive studies such as Strode and Barrett-Grant (2001) how large and widespread these effects are. The main aim of these studies seems to be identifying areas of human rights abuse that can be addressed by policy and legislative change, not measuring how extensive these problems are.

Studies that quantify disadvantage for children (especially orphans) can be used to suggest the impact of stigma but it is not always easy to assess what is causing these effects. If we want to understand more about the impact of stigma and related discrimination on children we need more systematic investigations. Longitudinal studies can be helpful in identifying causal effects, and comparing children across socio-economic boundaries may help us to unpack the relationships between stigma, orphanhood and poverty. We need to find ways of analysing the quantitative data from high-prevalence countries to analytically separate the effects of the pandemic itself (for example, parental bereavement, increased poverty) from the effects of HIV/AIDS-related stigma. Using multiple qualitative methods may enhance our understanding of the problem.

3.2.3 Hypothesis 1c: Stigma exacerbates material and psychosocial effects of the pandemic on support systems for children

In understanding the impact of stigma and discrimination on children, we need to understand its impact on their caregivers, whether these caregivers are biological parents or not, and whether they are HIV-positive or not. The literature on the effects of HIV/AIDS-related stigma on adults (reviewed in Deacon et al. 2005) can be drawn on in understanding what secondary effects AIDS-related stigma and discrimination might have on children.

As has been suggested in the case of race and sexual behaviour, stigmatisation of caregivers, particularly mothers, can have negative impacts on children (Rebhun 2004). Mawn (1999) interviewed parents of HIV-positive children and highlighted the impact of stigma and isolation on their lives. Another study used in-depth interviews to explore the extent and effects of courtesy stigma experienced by grandparents caring for HIV-positive grandchildren in the US (Poindexter 2002). In sub-Saharan Africa there is a significant trend towards older people becoming caregivers for children, so these issues are receiving some attention.

Stigma and related discrimination can reduce the capacity of families and communities to provide adequate material support for children. Stigma and discrimination towards PLWHA and their families can result in the reduction of income for households through unfair dismissal, or loss of patronage in restaurant or trading businesses (Dodge &

Khiewrord 2005; John & Sainsbury 2003; Strode & Barrett-Grant 2001). Social isolation of PLWHA and their families is common. PLWHA or their families may choose to resign their jobs or move towns rather than face stigma or discrimination (Chase & Aggleton 2001; Silver Pozen 1995). A large proportion of fathers in studies at Groote Schuur and Red Cross hospitals (Strode & Barrett-Grant 2001) abandoned their families after the mother was diagnosed HIV-positive. The loss of a father has negative economic implications for the household (Case & Ardington 2004).

HIV-positive parents may fail to seek treatment for themselves when they need it because of denial, internalisation and expectations of stigma (Gewirtz & Gossart-Walker 2000), resulting in premature loss of earning power and death. Parents who cannot access proper treatment and support networks because of the consequences of disclosing their own status may not be in a position to care properly for their children. Parents who have not disclosed their own status may also choose not to formula-feed their children as this might be interpreted as indicating that they have HIV/AIDS (Skinner 2002). Accepting HIV/AIDS-related assistance from NGOs or the state can be a form of disclosure, and may therefore be problematic for some families (Mills 2004). Also, non-recipients may be jealous of the special treatment received by HIV-affected families in an environment of scarcity. This may exacerbate ill-feeling towards families who accept HIV/AIDS-related assistance.

In situations in developing countries where public health facilities are inadequate and overstretched, families are the primary caregivers to PLWHA. Poverty creates a context in which difficult decisions about resource allocation have to be made at a household level. AIDS-related stigma may have become a more socially acceptable justification for discrimination than poverty in allocation of resources in some high-prevalence areas like Zambia (Bond et al. 2003). Stigma and discrimination can compromise the treatment and care of PLWHA within the home (Aggleton 2001). There is some evidence that women are more likely to be badly treated than children and men in households (Bharat & Aggleton 1999 and Castro et al., 1998a, 1998b in Aggleton et al. 2001). Reduced care for women will have a knock-on effect on children, however, as women remain the primary caregivers of children.

In addition to parental unavailability through illness or death, stigma and related discrimination can reduce the capacity of parents and communities to provide adequate psychosocial support to their children (Leslie et al. 2002). Increased relative poverty would also be a source of parental stress. Internalisation of stigma can lead to low self-esteem and depression in parents (Berger et al. 2001; Hackl et al. 1997), social withdrawal or exclusion caused by stigma is associated with chronic depression and loss of support networks, especially in HIV-positive women (Ingram & Hutchinson 1999; Lichtenstein et al. 2002). Fear of stigma or discrimination can exacerbate feelings of anxiety and hopelessness (Bogart et al. 2000). Parental depression can have serious negative effects on children (Wolchik & Sandler 1997), and can reduce the ability of parents to help their children cope with the parental diagnosis and its consequences, as well as meet their own developmental needs (Reyland et al. 2002).

In conclusion, HIV/AIDS-related stigma can have serious effects on the emotional, physical and material wellbeing of caregivers of children affected or infected by HIV/AIDS. This directly and indirectly affects the children who are in their care. There is an increasing body of work on parenting and HIV/AIDS in wealthier countries, which is highlighting issues of stigma. The effects of stigma on caregiver and other support systems now need to be recognised as critical variables in the literature on material and psychosocial effects of the pandemic on children in developing countries.

3.3 Hypothesis 2: HIV/AIDS-related stigma towards children is framed within different social discourses

Understanding the content of HIV/AIDS-related stigma towards children is important because different forms of stigmatisation may have different effects on children, and some may be more intense than others.

3.3.1 Hypothesis 2a: HIV/AIDS-related stigma towards adolescents is affected by discourses about sexual activity in children.

Stigmatising discourses are drawn into broader power dynamics in society, for example the attempt by adults to delay or control child (especially adolescent) sexual debut.

Ogden and Nyblade (2005) place children at the innocent end of their blaming continuum between guilt and innocence. While younger children who contracted HIV through birth or blood transfusion may not be blamed for having the disease, adolescents may be blamed for engaging in sexual intercourse or drug use, and thus bringing the disease upon themselves through 'immoral' actions. Campbell et al. (2005) suggest that stigma or gossip around HIV/AIDS is used by adults as a way of socially policing and punishing transgressive adolescent sexuality.

Figure 2: 'Innocence-to-guilt' continuum

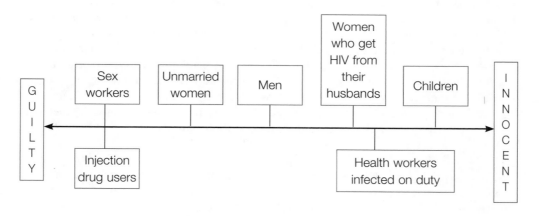

Source: Ogden & Nyblade 2005: 23

Adolescents are at high risk for contracting HIV: in high-prevalence communities, most new infections occur during adolescence (Venier & Ross 1997 in Leclerc-Madlala 2002). If gossip is one mechanism for adult control over adolescents, which seems likely, it is curious that adolescents also participate in this process. According to research on urban Zambian adolescents (Joffe & Bettega 2003), adolescents themselves engage in similar blaming discourses that link HIV/AIDS to promiscuity, sex for money and lack of self-control. Adolescent girls were particularly likely to be blamed for the spread of AIDS (even by other girls), through relationships with sugar daddies in order to get money; female sex workers were also blamed for spreading the disease; and in about 40 per cent of interviews, adolescent boys were blamed by other adolescents for not restraining their sexual desires.

It is difficult to change adolescent behaviours that put them at risk for HIV (Kaaya et al. 2002). There is still relatively little formal discussion of sexual matters between parents and children in places like South Africa (Brookes et al. 2004). Adolescents also subscribe to alternative discourses around sexual behaviour, for example the notion that being pregnant makes one a 'real' woman, or having many partners (or sexually-transmitted infections) is a sign of manhood. Youth sexual culture in much of sub-Saharan Africa is characterised by male dominance, high levels of sexual violence, widespread provision of sex for gifts from 'sugar daddies', and a pattern of younger women and girls having sex with older men (Leclerc-Madlala 2002). Many of these patterns of behaviour are condoned by parents who want their daughters to find a man, or are struggling for money at home (Kelly & Ntlabati 2002).

In conclusion, the intensity and nature of stigmatisation around HIV/AIDS is likely to vary considerably depending on the gender and extent of sexual experience of the child. Adolescents may well be more heavily stigmatised by adults than younger children for having HIV, or even for having HIV-positive parents, because of the assumption that they acquired HIV because they violated adult norms of sexual debut. Among adolescents themselves, however, engaging in sexual activity or even having STIs may have different and sometimes positive social meanings, particularly for boys.

3.3.2 Hypothesis 2b: HIV/AIDS-related stigma towards younger children is affected by discourses about poverty, streetchildren and orphanhood

Overt HIV/AIDS-related discrimination and stigma against children is becoming less common than stigmatisation of HIV-affected children for their poverty (Strode & Barrett-Grant 2001). Foster et al. (1997) found that Zimbabwean orphans faced stigmatisation based on orphan status or poverty, rather than the possibility that the parent died from AIDS. OVC in Zimbabwe were reportedly sometimes shy to interact with other children because they didn't have the good clothes owned by wealthier non-orphans (Mahati et al. 2006). Such children avoided going to church or playing with other children, and they felt that they were infrequently selected for participation in community youth programmes because of their poverty (Mahati et al. 2006). Research conducted in Zambia among children aged between 7 and 15 years revealed that children were being blamed for being 'orphans, being HIV positive, the fact that their parents have died from AIDS, being a "burden", or being street children' (Clay et al. 2003).

It is not surprising that HIV/AIDS-related stigma is often associated with stigma around orphanhood, lack of a formal home (being a street child) and poverty. There are four main ways in which poverty and stigma can be linked:
1. Poor people are more vulnerable to contracting HIV and developing symptoms of AIDS more quickly;
2. HIV infection in a household may lead to a cycle of increasing poverty as breadwinners become ill and die;
3. HIV and AIDS-related stigma is often linked to stigmatising beliefs around poverty (e.g. stigma towards street children); and
4. Poverty can be a reason for differential treatment of HIV-positive people within families.

Giese et al. (2003a) and Monasch and Boerma (2004) show how orphanhood is also associated with poverty, and a number of disadvantages for children. In a situation of poverty, families have to make difficult choices about spending scarce resources (Bond et al. 2003; Clay et al. 2003). AIDS-related stigma or orphanhood may be called on to justify the discrimination necessitated by poverty. This could be called resource-based stigma (Stein 2003b), or in fact household triage. The effects of HIV/AIDS-related stigma and poverty have to be seen in the context of other factors like loss of parental care or other forms of stigma in driving disadvantage for children.

Figure 3: Interactions between poverty, bereavement and HIV/AIDS stigma

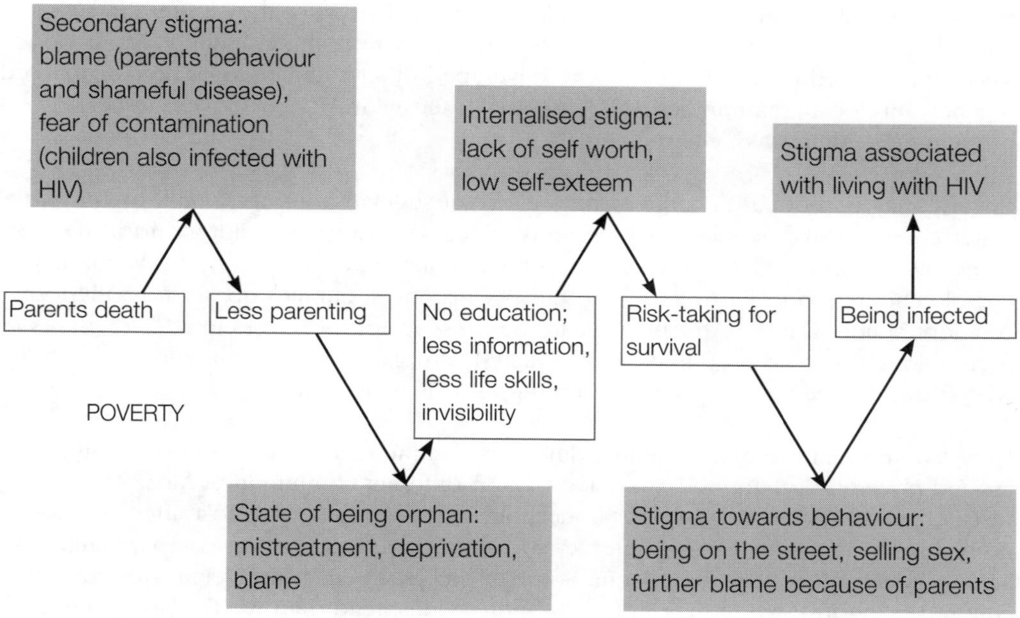

Source: Clay et al. 2003: 38

There is often an interaction between pre-existing forms of stigmatisation or prejudice (e.g. racism, sexism, homophobia) and later forms of disadvantage such as HIV/AIDS-related stigma. Research suggests that poverty has a huge impact on children, materially and emotionally (Brooks-Gunn et al. 1997 and Fitzgerald et al. 1995 in Stein 2003a). A history of poverty may thus make coping with stigma more difficult as well as making stigmatisation more likely. Taking the example of black children in the UK, Bernard sketches out the following possible interaction between child abuse and racism:

> In a context of societal devaluation, internalised narratives of racism will profoundly affect the way trauma is conceptualised, understood and named. Given the pervasive racism that structures black children and their families' lives, it is not surprising that there will be reluctance to publicly name some aspects of parental behaviour as abusive. (Bernard 2002: 248)

Unlike drug use, promiscuity and homosexuality, however, poverty and the absence of a parent have not been highly stigmatised in the past, especially in Africa where both have been widespread. Orphanhood and poverty could have been stigmatised in recent years more because they are acting as a marker of being affected by AIDS than because they are perceived as stigmatising in their own right (Webb 1997 in Ansell & Young 2004). Ansell and Young noted that stigmatisation of orphans was a more noticeable pattern in places like Lesotho where 'AIDS is more recent, less widespread and carries greater stigma' (2004: 6). When discussing 'layered stigma', we need to be clear about whether we are talking about a discourse that builds on existing stigmatising discourses, or a discourse in which one or more factors are actually serving as secondary markers for a more highly stigmatised issue.

Meintjes and Giese (2006) point out, however, that words for 'orphan' in indigenous South African languages like isiXhosa or seSotho are associated with a pre-AIDS stigma not because they imply lack of a biological parent but because they imply the lack of any adult carer: a child forsaken by society, a child with nothing, a child who is poor. The English word for orphan may have developed other stigmatised or non-stigmatised meanings in local communities, by being associated with AIDS or poverty relief programmes (Meintjes & Giese 2006).

Poverty may be both an incentive and a cause of stigmatisation for families who formally foster children. Such families may be represented as taking the children in for the money alone (Davids et al. 2006). And indeed some families may specifically choose to take in eligible children in order to get the grant. Because most families do not formally foster or adopt children in the African context, the presence of incentives like foster grants for non-biological caregivers (Meintjes et al. 2003) can play a role in stigmatising families who foster children, precisely because there is a financial reward.

It is also important to note potential differences in the relationship between stigma around poverty, orphanhood and HIV/AIDS in different communities. Most AIDS-related research in Africa focuses on poor households because these are most affected, most numerous and most in need of interventions, but there is a need to compare children across the socio-economic spectrum. Some of the experiences and 'characteristics' of children living in poverty may in fact be more widespread than we think. A study in Sao Paulo, Brazil (de Moura 2004), for example, compared the health-related concerns of relatively deprived street children, poor but housed adolescents and privileged adolescents. One of the interesting conclusions of that study (contrary to what was found by Swart-Krueger & Richter 1997) was that street children were no less concerned or more fatalistic about disease than poor or privileged children. However, it was not clear whether children from different socio-economic backgrounds could or would behave the same way. Poor children may be more constrained in acting on their beliefs.

Looking at patterns of stigmatisation across different socio-economic and epidemic contexts, taking any relevant cultural differences into account, can be instructive in establishing what the dynamic is between poverty, orphanhood and HIV/AIDS. This, especially within a longitudinal study design, may also help us to differentiate between the effects of stigma, poverty and HIV/AIDS on children. Researchers on child poverty have similarly concluded that to understand and address poverty better we need to know more about how distribution of resources within households affects children, and we need to have more longitudinal studies to make a better case for poverty advocacy choices (Hill & Smith 2003).

In conclusion, HIV/AIDS-related blaming discourses directed at younger children focus less on promiscuity than on poverty, orphanhood and other AIDS-related issues. Understanding the interactions between poverty, orphanhood, stigma and discrimination is particularly important because we need to know how to intervene most efficiently in poor, high-prevalence areas where HIV-affected children are suffering disadvantage.

If one provides food parcels to households, for example, will the food reach the most vulnerable children? To what extent is their disadvantage due to necessity-related household triage and to what extent are they being disadvantaged simply for their association with HIV/AIDS? Will they be further stigmatised for receiving food parcels (Mills 2004)?

However, as we note in the next section, younger children are often blamed for parental (especially maternal) sexual 'misbehaviour' that is assumed to be the cause of parental HIV status. This is probably a feature of HIV/AIDS-related courtesy stigma directed at both younger children and adolescents by peers.

3.4 Hypothesis 3: Children stigmatise each other

Given the prevalence of AIDS-related stigma in adults, and comparative research on other stigmatised diseases affecting children, it would be surprising if children themselves did not stigmatise each other. Children exhibit stigmatising attitudes towards people with other chronic diseases. A review of several studies on epilepsy (MacLeod & Austin 2003), suggests that adolescents in the USA do hold stigmatising views on epilepsy and three-quarters thought that this would result in discrimination against other adolescents with epilepsy (Austin et al. 2002 in MacLeod & Austin 2003). This may explain why although two-thirds of adolescents with epilepsy in a second study (Westbrook et al. 1992 in MacLeod & Austin 2003) did not report feeling stigmatised or discriminated against, less than half of the sample had disclosed publicly, and 70 per cent rarely or never spoke about their condition. Adolescents in another study (Westbrook et al. 1991 in MacLeod & Austin 2003) reported a similarly low rate of disclosure, significantly lower than for non-stigmatised chronic illnesses.

Some recent research has begun to look specifically at children's attitudes towards HIV-positive people in general (Castle 2004; Cossman 2004; Letamo 2004). This data will be examined further in the section on knowledge and stigma. In this section we will focus on whether children also stigmatise other children. Giese et al. found in their South African study that:

> Lindelwa…whose mother began to disclose publicly some time after testing HIV positive…was teased by peers at school that she too was HIV positive because she shared a bed with her mother – this despite the fact that she attended a school very active in AIDS education. Teachers in Umzimkulu described similarly how children talked openly about the fact that a parent had TB but that they are teased and laughed at by peers if they disclose that a parent has AIDS: 'They may say maybe their mother is a prostitute or their father doesn't handle himself in the right way.' If other children know that a child is HIV positive they 'might not want the child near them, they also might abuse the child with names'. Teachers in Gugulethu commented on their perceptions that 'even if a child's own sister died of AIDS, they will tease another child about HIV'. (2003b: 68–69)

In a 1994 study, Kuhn et al. (cited in Garvey 2003) found that in the absence of any educational interventions, only 17 per cent of the students said they would accept HIV-positive children into the classroom. Secrecy and stigma are also key problems for young people in Cote de Ivoire who cannot tell peers that they are HIV positive (Dago-Akribi & Cacou Adjoua 2004). Similar reluctance to disclose being affected by HIV in the family was noted among schoolchildren in two South African studies (Davids et al.

2006; Giese et al. 2003b). In Zambia, teachers reported to researchers that children who had lost both their parents had been taunted because of the perceived shame associated with a diagnosis of HIV (Baggaley et al. 1999). In Zimbabwe, some OVC reported being taunted by other children for their parents' death from HIV/AIDS, although other students dismissed reports that this was happening (Mahati et al. 2006).

In a Scottish study, a 13-year-old girl was not willing to disclose her mother's HIV status to her peers because of a (seemingly justified) fear that disclosure would lead to stigma and discrimination against her and her mother:

> Because, like, you get some really horrible people that will say nasty things about it and I really dinnae want that, because one of my other friends went and told this person, cos her mum is HIV, but I've never said anything, and this person told somebody else, an' she started being really horrible to her and saying that they didn't want to be friends wi' her any more an' some of the mums found out, so, like, they were being horrible to her mum, like ignoring her and things like that. So I dinnae want that to happen to me or my mum. (Cree et al. 2004: 15)

A 60-year-old grandparent of children orphaned by AIDS from Sudan made the following comment in one research study:

> I am facing a hard time. I am repelled from my family and the children keep on telling me about the relentless comments they hear from their peers because of their parents' illness and death. (International HIV/AIDS Alliance & Help Age International 2004: 8)

Quite a few research papers suggest that there is a gendered dimension to the nature of children's teasing at school. In the Scottish study, AIDS-related teasing (e.g. 'Yer ma's a mad jagger. She's riddled with fucking AIDS' [Cree et al. 2004:14]) illustrated that AIDS-related 'slagging' in Scotland is incorporated into a broader pattern of (male?) school-age teasing that involves 'mother-cussing' or insults directed at mothers and sisters (Renold & Barter 2002 in Cree et al. 2004). Cree et al. suggest that children take insults directed at family members very personally, and may thus be more vulnerable to courtesy stigma than adults.

Chase and Aggleton (2001) reported from Zambia that children whose parents had died as a result of HIV/AIDS, were sometimes taunted by other children saying, 'Your mother's a prostitute!' Strode and Barrett-Grant, quoting a woman living with HIV in Bloemfontein, provide a similar example from South Africa:

> Some children call to our kids, 'I'll give you your thin mother'. This happens to my child when he is playing with his friends especially if the hospice car comes by. They would say 'Your mother rides in a car that is ridden by people who have AIDS which means she has got AIDS too.' (2001: 17)

Some reported stigma may be because children may have fewer resources to offer. More than 500 respondents in five communities in SA and Namibia were surveyed in 1992–93 about what they think should happen to children orphaned by AIDS. Teenagers and elderly people, most likely to be dependent themselves, were the least likely to be sympathetic to orphans, while the poorest and most affluent households were the most sympathetic (Webb 1995).

In the light of this discussion about the cruelty of children to each other, it may be interesting to compare children's self-reports of experienced or expected stigma or discrimination from adults in general, guardians, and other children. In the Kanana township in South Africa, 16 per cent of the OVC aged 6–14 that were surveyed said that adults in the community did not support people living with HIV (Simbayi et al. 2006). A smaller proportion of children in this age group (10 per cent), said that they themselves were treated badly by their guardians: most (88 per cent) said they were not treated badly. An even lower proportion of children said that other children in the community (2.4 per cent) refused to play with them, and non-siblings in the household (5.3 per cent) treated them badly.

While older children aged 15–18 reported bad treatment by guardians (11.2 per cent of the sample) and different treatment of orphans by adults (18.3 per cent of the sample), there was a surprisingly high proportion of children (many of whom were orphans themselves) who felt that orphans received preferential treatment. Clearly, these questions are not probing the same issue across categories (adults in general, guardians, children at home, children in the community), so the answers are not comparable. But they do suggest that children in this sample may not be experiencing or reporting as much bad treatment from other children than they are from guardians and possibly from other adults.

In conclusion, children's stigmatisation of each other can have serious and negative effects on their wellbeing and even on their access to education. It also seems to be highly gendered in content, specific attention being paid to the status of the mother. Children tend to take familial insults very personally. It is not clear, however, whether children and young adults stigmatise more or less than do adults. It is also not clear whether stigmatisation and discrimination by children has more or less effect on other children than does stigmatisation and discrimination by adults.

3.5 Hypothesis 4: Children experience stigma differently depending on their stage of emotional and cognitive development

Adolescents are in a state of transition, embarking on their sexual careers (laden with proscription and tension), developing their adult identity, and very sensitive to peer norms (MacLeod & Austin 2003) and thus may be likely to both express and experience stigma more deeply than both adults or younger children. Younger children could also be vulnerable to stigma, however. They may be particularly likely to personalise experiences, making them very vulnerable to courtesy stigma because they would, for example, take insults against their mother personally (Cree et al. 2004). With a smaller frame of experiential references, younger children may also be more likely to normalise experiences, making them less likely to react against stigma and discrimination because they might perceive abuse as normal.[15]

There is an argument for looking specifically at children's responses to stigma (which can be understood as a stressor) because children are likely to perceive a stressor, its context, and their own ability to respond to it, differently from adults. It is necessary to understand how children experience and respond to stigma in order to reduce its impact on their development, health and wellbeing.

---

15 L Cluver, comments on this paper.

3.5.1 Understanding how children cope

One fruitful approach to understanding how children deal with stigma at different cognitive and emotional stages of development can be found in the coping literature. Eisenberg et al. (1997) use a broad definition of coping and emotional regulation that includes purposeful and unconscious attempts to directly regulate emotion (e.g. acceptance, denial, avoidance), the situation itself (e.g. problem-solving), and emotionally-driven behaviour (e.g. aggression). Clearly, children can be assisted by others (e.g. caregivers) in developing optimal coping skills (as the discussion above shows). The use of coping strategies changes with cognitive and emotional development. Individuals may favour specific coping mechanisms (temperament). The context of stressful events, including their salience and controllability, also affects children's response to it.

Eisenberg et al. define optimal coping or regulation as involving:

> flexible use of regulatory mechanisms, relatively high use of constructive modes of regulation such as activational control [the ability to initiate and maintain behaviour, particularly behaviours that are not pleasurable], attentional control (e.g., attention shifting and focusing), planning and problem solving, and moderately high use of inhibitory control. (1997: 47)

Lack of flexibility in response characterises both underregulation (where low use of regulation results in impulsive/resistant/acting-out behaviours) and over- or highly inhibited regulation (where consistent high use of inhibition control results in avoidant, fearful behaviour). Avoidant strategies may be more appropriate in uncontrollable situations (Eisenberg et al. 1997).

3.5.2 Emotional and cognitive coping strategies in young children and adolescents

Because of differences in blaming discourses around the mode of infection, children's stage of emotional and cognitive development, and environmental factors like family roles and expectations, stressors like stigma have variable effects on children of different ages. Peer support becomes increasingly important to children as they grow older: it acts as a forum for self-disclosure, advice and support, helping them deal with stressors (Eisenberg et al. 1997). Adolescents may thus suffer more than younger children if they are isolated from these sources of support and be at higher risk of low self-esteem if peers stigmatise them.

Research on children with cleft lips or palates suggests that even at primary school (age 7), however, lower-self esteem may be associated with social stigmatisation. At this age, even children without visible disability commonly have problems with peer acceptance and independence and may thus be vulnerable to stigmatisation (Broder & Strauss 1989).

Adolescence is a critical period for identity formation in which adolescents have a greater need to conform to peer norms (MacLeod & Austin 2003). Adolescents may therefore experience more conflict around feelings of difference than younger children.

> [I]n adolescence, the role models of identity and source of emotional dependency shift from parents to peers. The gang and the clique give adolescents the opportunity to practise trying on roles to see whether or to what extent they will fit them. Dependency on peers will give way to a mature identity and a sense of inner assurance. (Erikson 1959 in Reyland et al. 2002: 292)

Where adolescents have to carry the burden of secrecy around their parent's HIV status, or their own, they may distance themselves from their peers and thus hamper the process of identity development (Reyland et al. 2002).

The emotion-focused coping strategies favoured by adolescents may increase the distress associated with their own or parental illness, reducing their ability to cope with stigma as an additional stressor. As children get older, they use a greater variety of coping strategies and can recognise and avoid situations in which they cannot control themselves or the stressor. Older children employ fewer physical and material strategies (e.g. going out of the room) and more cognitive strategies (e.g. distraction, positive thinking).

This means that adolescents are more likely than younger children to use emotion-focused coping and thus try and avoid negative thoughts, a strategy that has been associated with greater distress than problem-focused coping or dual-focused coping (Worsham et al. 1997). A child's age at the time of diagnosis of terminal parental illness thus affects the adjustment of a child: adolescents have more problems adjusting than do younger children (Worsham et al. 1997).

Although older children are less likely to become overwhelmed in stressful situations, they are more likely to internalise negative experiences and information and may be more realistic in their self-perceptions and in perceptions of the intentions and beliefs of others (Eisenberg et al. 1997). In research on children with parents who have cancer, adolescents were found to have greater adjustment problems than younger children (Compas et al. 1994 cited in Forehand et al. 1998), perhaps because of more knowledge about illness or greater responsibilities in the family.

Because of social strictures around adolescents engaging in consensual sex, adolescents, especially young women, may experience greater AIDS-related stigmatisation than younger children (who are assumed to be innocent victims) or adults (whose sexual activity is socially sanctioned).

3.5.3   Ignorance, knowledge and stigma

Herek (2002) distinguishes between 'symbolic stigma' (moral judgements) and 'instrumental stigma' (social distancing or discrimination arising from fear of infection based on ignorance – to this one could add resource-based concerns like poverty, see Stein 2003b). Since ignorance of modes of transmission has been linked to increased stigma in a number of studies (Herek 2002; Kalichman & Simbayi 2003), it is appropriate to ask whether children express less stigma as they acquire more knowledge about disease in general and specific knowledge about transmission modes for HIV/AIDS.

The relationship between ignorance of transmission methods and stigmatising beliefs or discrimination is complex. Early approaches to researching stigma have been rightly criticised for focusing on stigmatising attitudes as the key cause of stigma (Parker & Aggleton 2003), but explaining stigma as an agent of social control by the powerful in society is, as we have seen, equally unsatisfactory. If stigma is a process of blaming and othering, based on fear, where does ignorance fit in?

Ignorance of the modes of transmission of HIV can certainly cause negative beliefs about and unfair discrimination against people infected or affected by HIV or AIDS. But is this necessarily stigma? Not all negative beliefs about disease (correct or incorrect) should be classified as stigma, because stigma is specifically about blaming and shaming. And ignorance can cause unfair discrimination without being associated with stigma at all. However, ignorance does not just cover the 'do not know', but also the 'do not want to know' – ignorance is not just a lack of knowledge, but a kind of knowledge that decides what is unknowable.

Thus, some instances of ignorance may be associated with moral judgement, and it may be difficult to identify which instances can thus be classified as stigma in our definition of it, except by seeing whether it is easy to shift them by providing knowledge. This kind of test would be complicated by the fact that provision of knowledge has been seen in very simplistic terms, in much HIV/AIDS education, as the provision of public health slogans in pamphlets. As Ogden and Nyblade (2005) report, people have complex questions, especially in high-prevalence areas – questions that need more intensive workshopping and discussion. Also, public health messages (for example, condoms prevent HIV transmission) are often based on the estimation of risk at an epidemiological level, whereas people make personal risk decisions using different kinds of criteria (for example, is there ANY risk of sex with condoms if their sex partners are HIV discordant?).

Also, some people living with HIV or AIDS may prefer to believe that they contracted the virus through casual contact because this reduces the stigmatising association between HIV transmission and sexual activity. Zuyderduin (2004) found, for example, that 10 per cent of the PLWHA she polled in Botswana believed that they had contracted the disease through contact with cups and utensils and not through sex.

When considering the relationship between ignorance, stigma and discrimination, therefore, it is critical to also consider the relationship between prevention messages, context of message source and recipient, reasons for holding specific beliefs, and mode of knowledge acquisition. People who believe that AIDS is caused by witchcraft, for example, may be less likely to believe, and therefore 'know', public health messages about prevention (see Kalichman & Simbayi 2004).

This rather complex debate about the relationship between knowledge and stigma needs to be overlaid with a debate about the relationship between children's knowledge acquisition and stigma. There is a small body of work on children's developmentally and culturally-influenced acquisition of knowledge about disease and its causality (Johnson et al. 1994; Peltzer & Promtussananon 2003), suggesting that children move slowly towards understanding biomedical models of disease.

There is, however, little research that critically explores the relationship between stigma, knowledge acquisition and emotional development in children. Research on children with epilepsy has shown that older adolescents had greater cognitive appreciation for the longer-term implications of having the chronic disease than younger children, and consequently a more negative perception of the disease (for example, its role in limiting social activities and causing isolation). This accounted for a lower reported health-related quality of life in older children, independently of disease duration (Devinsky et al. 1999).

There is some data on children's knowledge about HIV/AIDS transmission in sub-Saharan Africa. LoveLife's survey in 2000 found that 20 per cent of 12–13 year-olds sampled across South Africa had not even heard of HIV (Lee 2005). Brookes et al. (2004: 36) suggest that knowledge about HIV/AIDS transmission in 12–14 year-old South African children is deficient, for example, with only a quarter of their sample (n=740) believing HIV is transmitted through contaminated blood, a third believing HIV can be transmitted through sharing needles, and only half of their sample believing HIV can be transmitted through unprotected vaginal sex. A study of 11–14 year-olds in Western Cape schools showed that 22 per cent of students believed the virus could be transmitted by shaking hands (Lee 2005). Younger children showed a greater increase in knowledge and non-stigmatising attitudes than older children after an educational intervention in that study. Older children sometimes showed a decrease in knowledge and an increase in stigmatising attitudes after that intervention (Lee 2005).

Generally, one would expect to see an increase in knowledge about HIV/AIDS as children get older. Comparing the age categories 12–14 years and 15–18 years, young people in Zimbabwe's Chimanimani district showed an increase in knowledge about HIV/AIDS and its transmission (Gomo et al. 2006). This was followed by a slight decrease in knowledge in the category 19–24 years, perhaps because of information campaigns targeted at school-going children. This suggests that we cannot assume a direct relationship between age and knowledge about HIV/AIDS. It is also difficult to know how to interpret this kind of data, in the light of a study that suggests children's knowledge of disease processes, and not their ability to assess the correctness of key phrases, is the critical factor in assessment of their knowledge about HIV/AIDS. Children's knowledge of disease processes may not, unfortunately, be easily measurable in fixed-format questions (Obeidallah et al. 1993).

If one focuses on trends towards giving correct responses on key phrases, however, it may be possible to see whether this corresponds with a trend towards fewer stigmatising attitudes among young people, as it does in adults. In the Chimanimani study, stigmatising attitudes towards HIV-positive people seemed to increase when the age categories 15–24 years and 25+ years were compared. We were unable to see whether this related to a decrease in knowledge about HIV/AIDS from the published data (Gomo et al. 2006). Other studies have shown a variable trend – some finding that older people stigmatise less, and others that older people stigmatise more. In a research project examining HIV/AIDS-related stigma in South Africans in the Cape Town Metropolitan area using the CAPS and Cape Area Study (CAS) studies at the Centre for Social Science Research (CSSR), UCT, Maughan-Brown (work in progress) has found somewhat less intended discriminatory behaviour towards HIV-positive people being reported by young adults (15–23 years) than by older adults. Young adults also expressed less instrumental (risk-based) and symbolic (moral judgment-based) stigma than adults, although the comparison is possible on only two questions.

Most other surveys suggest higher levels of reported stigma among young adults than among adults. The Demographic and Health surveys (DHS) (see Table 1) in sub-Saharan Africa indicate similar or higher rates of stigmatising attitudes (lack of acceptance of PLWHA) in adolescents (15–19 years) than in all adults (15–49). Adolescents in Botswana, especially males, showed evidence of considerable stigmatisation towards adult PLWHAs (questions were not asked about peer stigmatisation). A large proportion of adolescents (aged 10–19) in the Botswana study expressed stigmatising attitudes towards people living with HIV/AIDS, about half saying that an HIV-positive teacher should not be allowed to teach and two-thirds saying that they would not buy goods from an HIV-positive shopkeeper (Letamo 2004). People aged between 10 and 25 (especially males) were significantly more likely than older adults to show stigmatising attitudes: they were over five times more likely to say they were not willing to care for an HIV-positive family member, about three times more likely to say that HIV-positive teachers should not teach, and two to three times more likely to say they would not buy goods from HIV-positive shopkeepers (Letamo 2003).

Table 1: Age-differentiated measures of stigma, from DHS surveys

Country	Accepting attitudes towards those living with HIV[*]					
	Percentage of sample population		Percentage of age group			
			15–19 years		15–49 years	
	Male	Female	Male	Female	Male	Female
Mozambique Demographic and Health Survey 2003	15	8	14	10	16	8
Tanzania HIV/AIDS Indicator Survey 2003–04	37	27	28	22	37	27
Zambia Sexual Behaviour Survey 2000	21	18	-	-	-	-
Zambia Demographic and Health Survey 2001–2002	15	9	14	8	16	9
Zambia Sexual Behaviour Survey 2003	29	24	-	-	-	24

Source: www.measuredhs.com
* This is a composite of four components, expressed as a percentage of the population sampled (some data expressed as a percentage of those who answered the question).

The complexity of exploring the relationship between developmental change, stigma and knowledge acquisition is illustrated by the lessons learned in work on prevention. Children have, and perhaps even more importantly, believe they have, less control over their circumstances than do adults. While adolescents have greater knowledge and understanding of illness than younger children, they also exhibit poorer judgement of personal risk than do adults and, in many cases, experience inadequate control over the circumstances of sexual encounter (Joffe & Bettega 2003). The likelihood that children will engage in unsafe sexual activity during adolescence because they cannot prevent it, or because they feel they are not at risk, places them at great risk for HIV infection, whatever their knowledge of prevention methods. Adolescent mothers-to-be show much lower rates of attendance at public antenatal clinics than older mothers-to-be (Letamo 2003). These factors place adolescents at a significant disadvantage compared to both younger children and adults in preventing and treating HIV infection.

In conclusion, measuring children's knowledge about HIV/AIDS or attitudes towards PLWHA, is difficult. It is often difficult to interpret the results, even when one has asked clear questions in good questionnaires. Testing knowledge by asking fixed-format questions can give us very limited information about the child's contextual grasp of the information. It is also difficult to increase knowledge by simply providing factual information, because knowing something depends on a range of factors including trust in the source of the information, and the cognitive ability and practical skills required to apply the information in the real world. Knowledge does not translate directly into attitudes or behaviour.

3.5.4 Other factors that affect children's experience of stigma

There are of course a number of factors that affect experience of stigma and other stressors besides the age of the child, the child's knowledge about HIV/AIDS, and his or her general stage of emotional or cognitive development. These factors include the degree to which the child is affected by HIV/AIDS (infected, caregiver ill or dead, relative ill or dead, etc.), the level of symptoms evident in the ill person and the child's perception of the seriousness of their illness, the ill person's cognitive impairment and emotional distress related to the illness (although this may be less important than the level of consequent family responsibility stress that devolves on mainly adolescent girls, see Worsham et al. 1997), the gender of the child and infected adult, the level of psychosocial support received by the child (Wild et al. 2005), and the disclosure status of infected relatives, as keeping parental status secret is a known stressor (Murphy et al. 2002).

Multiple social stressors affect children in high-prevalence areas like southern Africa, given for example that children may be poor, and orphaned as well as subject to AIDS-related stigma. AIDS is also not the only stigmatised illness affecting children, and some of these illnesses may be further stigmatised through their association with HIV/AIDS. Children consider a range of health concerns depending on their perceived severity and likelihood of contraction: in one study, adolescents in Sao Paolo feared AIDS and cancer most of all diseases (de Moura 2004).[16]

Strode and Barrett-Grant (2001) suggest that, like adults, children's experience of stigma and discrimination is gendered: AIDS is perceived as a female problem, girls do more home care work, and are perceived as responsible for controlling male sexuality. HIV-positive mothers rather than fathers may be targeted in school playground insults. In the family, age as well as gendered roles and expectations mediate a child's experience of having HIV-positive parents or siblings. Adolescents with sick parents (especially girls) are more likely to be information providers for others, and to receive certain kinds of companionship from family members (e.g. discussing the mother's illness with her), both of which tend to increase distress (Worsham et al. 1997).

Research on siblings of disabled children in the US (Lobato et al. 1987) suggested that sisters experienced greater restrictions on their time than brothers because they were expected to act as caregivers for their siblings. But perhaps because they had an active and clearly defined role in the family as a result, younger sisters of disabled children suffered less depression than younger brothers who experienced considerably reduced demands and expectations from parents. Older sisters of disabled children, who may have wanted greater freedom, suffered the highest rates of depression, anxiety and role tension.

3.6 Conclusion

In conclusion, although there are some protective effects of age in dealing with stressors, the greater knowledge, insight and vulnerability to peer opinion that comes with age, and the greater stigmatisation of HIV infection associated with sexual activity, tends to disadvantage adolescents both in being recipients of, and in coping with, AIDS-related stigma. Younger children affected by HIV/AIDS may, however, be more likely to

---

16 Given the highly stigmatised nature of cancer in the past, it is interesting that American mothers now frequently use cancer as a cover for their more highly stigmatised AIDS diagnosis (Ingram & Hutchinson 1999).

experience stigma and discrimination as normal and as personal,[17] and may therefore be vulnerable to internalisation thereof. Other factors such as the experience of AIDS-related illness and gendered expectations of children's roles in families need to be explored in order to fully understand the differential experience of stigma by children.

---

17 L Cluver, comments on this paper.

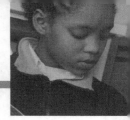

CHAPTER 4

Recommendations

4.1 Recommendations for research

Children are mainly perceived as problematic or needy by service agencies and governments if they do not have material necessities like food, homes and schooling, if their parents are dead or absent, or if they engage in externalising behaviours. Adult discourses about children that emphasise their innocence and purity on the one hand, and their resilience on the other, as well as the notion that the main task of support services is caring for mothers (for example as direct victims of domestic violence), allowing the benefits of support to filter down to children, have been used to explain the relative lack of attention paid to children's experiences of domestic violence (Caplan 2002).

These discourses seem to play a role in explaining the pattern of research and intervention on children affected by HIV/AIDS and HIV/AIDS-related stigma, which shows considerable divergence from the adult literature on AIDS-related stigma. Not many studies systematically investigate the experiences of stigma and discrimination of children affected by HIV/AIDS (although child-centred research seems to be a growing trend), and even fewer explore the experiences of HIV-positive children or the degree to which children stigmatise each other.

Specific research on HIV/AIDS-related stigma and children is minimal, and it tends to follow specific trajectories depending on the age of the subject. Research and intervention on AIDS-related stigma in adults seems to be concerned primarily with identifying stigmatising attitudes HIV-negative people hold about PLWHA. Research on adolescents focuses on the relationship between ignorance and early sexual debut or high-risk sexual behaviour, and research on younger children asks whether stigma affects disclosure or psychosocial adjustment after parental bereavement.

Stigma is most likely to be discussed in the literature on psychosocial effects of the pandemic on children, while discrimination is most likely to be discussed in the literature on material effects of the pandemic. This creates an unnecessary and artificial separation between the material and psychosocial effects stigma and discrimination have on children. Much of this research compares the material or psychosocial problems faced by (AIDS) orphans to those faced by non-orphans or other orphans. In high prevalence and impoverished communities, however, children in all three categories may experience similar problems, including stigmatisation associated with HIV/AIDS.

Most research on the psychosocial effects of HIV/AIDS on children presents stigma as an explanation for disadvantage or difference without specifically investigating it. Qualitative research on stigma and discrimination is good at enumerating the kinds of effects AIDS-related stigma and discrimination can have on children (Clay et al. 2003; Strode & Barrett-Grant 2001), but it is difficult to do any analysis on this data to determine how widespread the problem is and how it relates to other factors.

4.2 Research questions

Our previous work (Deacon et al. 2005) highlighted several critical areas of research on stigma in general.

4.2.1   The nature and extent of stigmatising beliefs:

- The content of stigmatising beliefs in a variety of social contexts;
- The extent to which stigmatising beliefs are held (in the general public) and supported (by media, prominent figures and so on) in society;
- The relationship between AIDS-related stigma and other forms of prejudice (e.g. racism, sexism) or social marginalisation (e.g. poverty).

4.2.2   The effects of stigma and related discrimination:

- The occurrence of discrimination related to stigma in different social contexts;
- Degree of stigmatisation and discrimination expected by infected and affected people;
- Degree of internalisation of stigmatising beliefs by infected and affected people;
- Effects of stigma and discrimination (experienced and expected) on infected and affected people.

The discussion above suggests that we also need more quantitative and qualitative empirical research on the nature and effects of stigma and discrimination on children, tracking decision-making processes and mapping the extent of the problem in households, schools and health care contexts. We need to understand the relationship between different kinds of stigma, discrimination and general disadvantage experienced by children affected by HIV/AIDS in order to determine which issues are most critical to address (e.g. AIDS-related stigma, poverty, access to services). We need to know more about how children themselves experience and practise stigma and discrimination, and about the moderating and mitigating factors affecting their responses. However, there are many challenges facing us because research on stigma is difficult, and research on children is particularly challenging and different from research on adults.

4.3   Choosing appropriate research methods

4.3.1   The research context

Research on stigma is affected by stigma. Many children and/or their caregivers will be HIV-positive without knowing their status, or, if they do, will be reluctant to reveal the fact to their communities or to researchers. In a setting up a study of the experiences of HIV-negative children of HIV-positive parents in Scotland, researchers found it difficult to recruit people for the study, especially the already stigmatised black and Asian ethnic minorities (Cree et al. 2004). Even in high-prevalence areas, South African researchers on experiences of children affected by HIV/AIDS have opted not to mention HIV/AIDS in materials provided to research participants because of the fear that stigmatisation of the condition may skew participation and responses (Cluver 2003).

Research on children, especially sick children, also raises ethical and communication considerations. There are various texts on how to ethically ensure children's participation, seek meaningful informed consent from children, ensure confidentiality and anonymity, and avoid stigma (Macklin 1992; Schenk & Williamson 2005). Some of the issues around obtaining parental consent in the South African context are described in Mathews et al. (2005).

Perhaps because of ethical and communication difficulties, much research on children continues to rely on behavioural observation and adult reports of children's feelings and behaviour. Hill and Smith (2003) and Giese et al. (2003b) highlight the importance of child participation in research processes, and noted in particular contrasting reports of stigma and discrimination from children and their caregivers. Other researchers have noted that parental report (or reports by other adults) may be an inaccurate measure of children's perception and experience of stigma (MacLeod & Austin 2003; Pfeffer et al. 2000).

Research into disability-related stigma has suggested that parental report may be systematically skewed by the need to present a self-protective public face to healthcare and welfare service providers (Green et al. 2005). Studies on racism suggest a similar trend towards underreporting by adults (in this case, teachers) of stigma and discrimination experienced by children (Donald et al. 1995). Interestingly, one study comparing illness experience after cancer treatment found significant correlations between child and parental reports of peer rejection in school (Eiser et al. 1995).

Psychosocial distress in children may also be under-reported by carers. Comparing children whose parents died of cancer or committed suicide, Pfeffer et al. found that children of parents who committed suicide reported significantly more depressive symptoms than other children, but their caregivers did not report the extent of the problem (Pfeffer et al. 2000). Parents, who may rely on their adolescent children's support, may underestimate their problems and needs. A study on children of parents with cancer found that, compared to children's self-reports, parents significantly underreported anxiety and depression in adolescent children but not in younger children (Welch et al. 1996 in Worsham et al. 1997).

There is also a power dynamic between children and adults (as researchers) that affects research results on sensitive topics like sexuality. Children may find it difficult to report sexual behaviour openly to adults or in the presence of caregivers. A southern and eastern African study (Pattman & Chege 2003) showed how adults' moralising discourses around pre-marital or adolescent sex, group dynamics and gender identities skews and silences adolescent reporting of their sexual behaviour. These problems can be partially addressed by treating children as experts on their own sexuality, encouraging non-judgemental data collection. Researchers could benefit from collecting data from mixed-sex and single-sex groups as well as from diaries (Pattman & Chege 2003). More participatory, narrative research methods could also be beneficial. Work on drug abuse suggests that adolescent self-report becomes less reliable as use of more stigmatised substances is being reported (Percy et al. 2005).

4.3.2   Using survey instruments to measure a child's experience of stigma

Although the experience of stigma may cause internalising problems such as depression and low self-esteem, measuring internalising and externalising problems may not be the best or only measure of the effects of AIDS-related stigma on the experience of children whose parents have HIV/AIDS. Not all studies find elevated risk of distress and maladjustment in children of parents with serious medical illness, and if they do, it is not always clear whether these increased levels of distress and maladjustment exceed clinical criteria, although they do in some studies (Worsham et al. 1997). Worsham et al. (1997) argue that studies of internalising and externalising problems in children (which dominate the literature on coping) should be accompanied by research into problems in adaptive functioning in peer relationships, school performance and developmentally appropriate activities.

In a study on Kenyan street children (Ayuku et al. 2003), standardised measures of health, nutrition, medical status and temperament were combined with Maastricht Social Network Analysis (MSNA) instrument, observation, key informant interviews and focus groups. The MSNA instrument is a qualitative instrument based on an hour's semi-structured interview that measures the structure and supportive function of a person's social networks. It was developed to understand and address the social integration of adults with chronic illness, but was recently used with some success in the Kenyan study (Ayuku et al. 2003). This kind of instrument could help us to understand the impact of social stigma or discrimination on the functioning of children. This would be particularly interesting in exploring the impact of 'gossip' on children. Gossip is regularly mentioned by both children and adults as a negative consequence or enactment of stigma (Clay et al. 2003; Cluver work in progress; Mills 2004; Strode & Barrett-Grant 2001). But it is difficult without some understanding of the value of social networks to assess what the cost of gossip might be. This might be accompanied by an economic analysis of the value of social networks.

Given the difficulty of self-report as a valid measure of stigmatising attitudes towards others, and the critical role of stigmatised people's experience of stigma in determining its effects (Deacon et al. 2005), one positive shift in the literature is the development of scales to measure expected (perceived) stigma in children and their caregivers (Austin et al. 2004). This follows some work done on measuring internalised and expected stigma in adults (Berger et al. 2001; Harvey 2001; Ritsher et al. 2003; Ross & Rosser 1996; Zickmund et al. 2003).

Quality of life studies designed for children with chronic disease can help measure the impact of disease-related stigma on quality of life (Cramer et al. 1999). This study suggested that experience of stigma had a large and negative effect on quality of life of children with epilepsy, explaining 22 per cent of the variance in the overall score. Poverty, greater severity and longer duration of illness, and attendance at special education classes were all associated with greater experience of stigma (Devinsky et al. 1999).[18]

More work could be done on adapting and verifying such scales to research African children's responses to AIDS-related stigma and other forms of stigma, including internalisation and expected stigma and discrimination. Lessons learned from testing adult stigma measures in Tanzania may need to be applied when adapting and testing scales for children (Tanzania Stigma-Indicators Field Test Group 2005).

Blaming attitudes and knowledge around HIV/AIDS have traditionally been measured in quantitative studies with adults by providing stigmatising statements with which respondents are required to agree or disagree, presenting fixed-format options or coding replies into fixed-format options. However, it is difficult to investigate children's experiences of stigma using direct questions. Some children have difficulty in understanding the questions, in engaging with abstract reasoning (especially younger children), and in disagreeing with what the peer group believes, or what the adult researcher is perceived to believe. Researchers should also be aware that giving incorrect options in questions about transmission modes or non-discriminatory statements may encourage children to adopt such knowledge and opinions.[19]

---

18 The stigma associated with special education, and severe epilepsy, could also have been due to secondary disclosure.
19 L Nyblade, personal communication.

There are often differences between children's knowledge measured by true-false questions (where 50 per cent of random answers could be correct), and open-ended questions. In a South African study, Lee (2005) found that children answered the same question about HIV transmission differently when they were formatted and phrased slightly differently. Obeidallah et al. (2003) found that children's responses to true-false or other limited-choice format questions were inconsistent with their responses to more open-ended questions in interviews. This was because the children often interpreted the meaning of the options in the fixed-choice questionnaires differently to adults (for example, understanding a dirty needle as a needle that had been stuck in dirt rather than as a needle that has had blood on it). So questions could be answered 'correctly' in fixed-choice surveys but the child may not actually be able to act on that knowledge correctly because the information has been misunderstood. Alternatively, questions could be answered 'incorrectly', but a child may be developing a sophisticated understanding about how biological disease processes operate.

4.3.3 Using multiple methods to investigate children's experience of stigma

To complement empirical studies which compare the functioning of groups of children on standard psychosocial measures or adapted stigma instruments, it may also be useful to conduct systematic qualitative and quantitative investigations of children's experiences of stigma with children. Increased use of multi-method research techniques has been called for in research on AIDS (Ackeroyd 1997 in Ansell & Young 2004) and stigma (Deacon et al. 2005). In the case of stigma research in children, this may be particularly important:

> Qualitative research methods may be better suited to uncovering the subtleties and complexities of how adolescents with epilepsy experience stigma and how it affects their lives… [For example, researchers could] ask a participant to tell a story about having epilepsy. (MacLeod & Austin 2003: 112)

Open-ended questions (which can be coded by researchers in an interview situation) may be more useful and more ethical than fixed-format self-report questions in measuring knowledge and attitudes among children. Although this reduces anonymity, even on an anonymous survey adolescents may struggle to express feelings of difference from peers because peer group identification is so important to them (MacLeod & Austin 2003). Worsham et al. (1997) make the case for using semi-structured interviews rather than self-report questionnaires when investigating coping strategies in children and adolescents, because the interviews can be more sensitive to children's individual differences. But they note that interviews can underreport coping strategies because children do not volunteer more than a few strategies themselves, and may need to be provided with a range of examples.

Qualitative methods for researching children's attitudes need to go beyond the interview. Non-verbal communication is a very important research tool with children. Pictures and drawings can be useful in measuring children's attitudes (for example, Klepsch 1982). Dolls have also been used for research with children (see Greene 1980 for a review of their use in racism studies). Clay et al. (2003) had considerable success (especially with the older children) getting Zambian children to draw stigmatising or discriminatory situations or perform dramatic sketches to illustrate them, after examples had been discussed with them. Clacherty and Kushlick (2004) used pictures and puppets with young children (3–6 years) while doing research for the Takelani Sesame television programme, which deals with HIV/AIDS and stigma. Both setting up of environments for questions and ranking of options were achieved with pictures. Children were also asked to draw pictures to help explain their responses to a question. The researchers emphasised the importance of designing age-appropriate research tools, dividing children into small, age-appropriate groups, running groups early in the day before children became tired, varying pace and activity to keep energy levels high, observing how children behaved to test emotional responses, keeping questions very concrete, and repeating questions throughout a session to enable triangulation of responses (Clacherty & Kushlick 2004).

Disability researchers have been particularly active in highlighting the importance of open-ended discussions, researcher identity, empathy and a trusting relationship between researcher and research participant when addressing stigmatised issues. Where a person feels highly stigmatised, or where researchers wish to explore experiences of stigmatisation, it may be useful for the researcher to have a similarly stigmatised identity or experience themselves. This may result in shared truths being constructed, but these shared truths may be more valuable in understanding the experience of the stigmatised community than the public 'coping' face that people may present to an outsider (Green et al. 2005). Speaking from both personal and professional experience, Hinshaw (2004) argues that quantitative methods should be blended with narrative accounts of children's experiences (in his case, children with mentally disordered parents) to reduce silencing, framing research questions and addressing the needs of the child.

4.3.4   Sample sizes and study design

Much of the current research on stigma and children can only sketch broad trends and provide examples of kinds of stigma and discrimination experienced by children partly because the best data is collected through individual or small-group qualitative work rather than through large surveys. Only a few studies (Clay et al. 2003; Strode & Barrett-Grant 2001) have systematically tried to investigate the experiences of large numbers of children faced by HIV/AIDS stigma, although quite a few studies touch on the issue using much smaller samples. Giese et al. (2003b) is an excellent example of a large qualitative study on children and HIV which combines child participatory research activities, interviews, focus group discussions and observation.

How do we link good qualitative work to meaningful quantitative data? Data collection using open-ended discussions rather than direct questions does not of course preclude the possibility of quantifying the results, but large interview samples may cost more to obtain than large questionnaire samples. More general surveys on the effects of the pandemic on children (Makame et al. 2002) could include more stigma-related variables to test the generalisability of the qualitative stigma research (Cluver, work in progress), but careful attention needs to be given to designing appropriate and useful questions on stigma for such surveys.

There are certainly benefits to analysing larger samples. Commenting on studies of children's coping around serious parental illness, Worsham et al. (1997) argued for larger sample sizes to enable researchers to analyse moderator variables with reasonable statistical confidence. They felt that more longitudinal studies were required to assess the nature of long- versus short-term adjustment and to track changes in adjustment over the course of parental illness in a prospective rather than retrospective manner. A similar point was made in regard to research on effects of parental bereavement on children (Lutzke et al. 1997). Cross-sectional studies may mask the true relationship between coping strategies and emotional distress: more distress may lead to a greater reliance on emotion-focused coping, rather than the other way around (Worsham et al. 1997).

Longitudinal studies may help in identifying factors that increase vulnerability in a child's lifetime. We have noted above that research on the effects of AIDS-related stigma on children suffers from the lack of a clearly defined control group. AIDS-related stigma and discrimination can affect not only children orphaned by AIDS, but also children whose HIV-positive caregivers or family members are sick, and children who are thought to be HIV-positive, or who are HIV-positive but whose parents are not.

In the absence of an easy definition of which children are going to be most affected by HIV/AIDS, and in areas where most children will be affected in some way, it may be pointless to search for a traditional control group. Even if we could find a control group, simply comparing the situation of affected and less affected children in cross-sectional study designs is not going to definitively identify the reasons for disadvantage. A better approach may be to focus on reasonably large samples, use longitudinal study designs, and to collect enough data on individual children to understand degrees of vulnerability, and to aim towards understanding whether stigma increases vulnerability, and in what ways it does so.

Wild et al. (2005) and other researchers have already discussed the importance of understanding the moderating and mediating factors that affect adjustment after parental diagnosis, illness or death or the child's contraction of HIV. Using age-appropriate qualitative and quantitative measures, researchers could gather some measures of children's knowledge, attitudes, behaviours and internalisation or experiences of stigma, together with information about factors that could affect their vulnerability to HIV/AIDS and the effects of HIV/AIDS-related stigma. These factors would include:

- **The child's living environment:** access to food, education, healthcare in the normal course of events, and how this has been affected by HIV/AIDS or associated poverty;
- **The direct effects of HIV/AIDS illness:** for example, whether the child is infected, caregiver ill or dead (gender is important), friend or relative ill or dead, and so on, the level of symptoms evident in the ill caregiver or child, the child's perception of the seriousness of the illness, and the ill caregiver or child's cognitive impairment and emotional distress related to the illness;
- **Secondary effects of the illness on the family:** for example, the level of family responsibility stress that devolves on the child, and how this is gender- or age-differentiated,
- **Characteristics of the child:** for example, the gender of the child, the child's age, the capacity of the child to cope with stressors (internal or external locus of control, level of knowledge, religious beliefs, and self-esteem);
- **Support available to the child:** for example, the level of psychosocial support received by the child (Wild et al. 2005), grief and depression in caregivers or family members; and
- **Extent of exposure to HIV/AIDS stigma and discrimination:** including that associated with other forms of prejudice such as race and gender, the child's interpretation thereof, the disclosure status of the child or infected caregivers, and so on.

Who should be researched? In the preceding discussion, we have suggested that orphans, or children orphaned by AIDS, should not be the sole focus of research on stigma and children. We have also suggested that both wealthy and poor children should be researched in order to help us assess the effects of poverty. A question that remains is whether researchers should focus more on younger children or on adolescents. Work on behavioural risks in the prevention arena initially focused on adolescents but the intervention strategy is increasingly moving towards a focus on the more easily influenced pre-adolescents, catching their attention before behaviour patterns are set.

Given adolescents' greater insight into the consequences of disease, higher risk of distress associated with illness, greater vulnerability to peer opinion and more intense stigmatisation than younger children, it may be advisable to focus some stigma-related research and intervention on adolescents infected and affected by HIV/AIDS, and the pre-adolescent group. There is already a large body of research on knowledge and behaviour in adolescents – we need more qualitative studies investigating older children's attitudes towards people living with HIV/AIDS, factors affecting disclosure, experiences of stigma and discrimination, and their responses to stigma and discrimination.

At the same time, it is critical to explore the consequences of normalising behaviours in younger children, which may increase the impact of internalisation of stigma on them.[20] By understanding experiences of stigma in both adolescents and pre-adolescents, researchers may be able to suggest ways in which interventions can both mitigate the effects of stigma on adolescent health-seeking, for example, and prepare pre-adolescents to cope better with HIV/AIDS-related issues in adolescence.

4.4   Recommendations for interventions

This study did not review interventions for children that might reduce HIV/AIDS-related stigma, and therefore the comments in this section are preliminary to such a review. This discussion seeks to raise issues about interventions that arise from the preceding discussion on research.

4.4.1   Should interventions target OVC?

Programmes addressing the impact of the AIDS pandemic on children have been more integrated, holistic and broad-ranging than those for adults. Programmes for children tend to take the child's material and household circumstances into account, whereas most programmes for adults have focused on prevention, treatment and care. However, most programmes for addressing the needs of children in the context of the AIDS pandemic still focus on orphans (Meintjes & Giese 2006; Richter et al. 2004).

In order to understand the impact on and experience of HIV/AIDS-related stigma in children, researchers need to disentangle the effects of AIDS-related stigma from the effects of other forms of stigma, caregiver illness and death, impoverishment, and other factors. Researchers try and understand how important stigma is in shaping the experiences of children affected by HIV/AIDS, what the consequences are for health and wellbeing, and how these impacts are being exacerbated or mitigated in various contexts. Along with more monitoring and evaluation of intervention programmes, this kind of research can help us design better interventions.

Although researchers may seek to identify which children are affected or infected by HIV/AIDS, it is debatable whether interventions should target specific groups of children affected by HIV/AIDS (such as children orphaned by AIDS). When conducting research to identify changing patterns in children's welfare (the epidemiological viewpoint) it is useful to establish what makes children vulnerable and to compare categories of

---

20 L Cluver, comments on this paper.

high vulnerability to categories of lower vulnerability. This approach is less useful in identifying *groups* of children who need assistance (the programmatic viewpoint). Appropriate assistance must be made available to all children who need it, whatever he reason they might have for needing it. Williamson et al. (2004) thus argue for a 'firewall' between definitions created for quantitative research purposes and for the purposes of policy and program implementation.

Is it possible to separate research and intervention terminology in this way? Even using terms like 'AIDS orphans', 'orphans and vulnerable children' (OVC) and 'children affected by HIV/AIDS' (CABA) in research work can be stigmatising (Bray 2003) and objectifying (Richter et al. 2004). That is why researchers reject such terms, or their abbreviations. Perhaps more significantly, we know that targeting specific groups for aid may further stigmatise them (Giese et al. 2003b). Even where children's problems may be caused by a specific factor, naming that factor may be stigmatising. Using a broader comparable example, even though epidemiologically it is true that having more (unprotected) sex puts one at greater risk of contracting HIV, it is unfortunate that the association of HIV/AIDS with greater sexual activity in public health programmes (for example, the ABC) has led to a stigmatising association of AIDS with promiscuity.

In the case of orphans, who are often targets of child-related interventions, it has been shown that they are often not at greater risk of disadvantage than non-orphans. Researchers have argued that children orphaned by AIDS (who have been the target of many HIV/AIDS-related interventions) actually experience many of the same problems as other poor children in high-prevalence areas. We thus need to provide services to all needy children in an equitable manner, without privileging orphans or foster children (Giese et al. 2003b). In a study on educational access using household survey data, Ainsworth and Filmer (2002) also found that orphan status was not a good predictor of educational enrolment in all countries. In countries with lower orphan than non-orphan enrolment, this was sometimes due to greater poverty in households with orphans, and sometimes to factors associated with orphanhood. They concluded that orphan status was not a good targeting criterion for improving educational access in most countries. General poverty relief, they said, will help poor orphans along with other poor children.

Even where orphans, for example, may be at a higher risk of experiencing certain kinds of problems than non-orphans (e.g. lower school attendance), targeting interventions exclusively at orphans may cause resources to be concentrated on the wrong issue (e.g. orphanhood rather than low school attendance). Similarly, profiling 'typical AIDS cases' as male, homosexual or drug-abusing in the early days of the epidemic was epidemiologically correct at the time, but it sometimes caused doctors in the US to miss the opportunity of correctly diagnosing cases in non-typical women. It also helped to stereotype gay men as disease carriers, and to distract attention from risk behaviours in which heterosexuals also engaged (Watney 1996). Profiling of drug mules (international smugglers) can similarly be counter-productive for anti-drug smuggling interventions, as customs officials start to ignore categories of people (e.g. old white women) as low risk, and these categories are recruited as the new drug mules.

Focusing on orphans and foster children can divert resources from other needy children. In South Africa, for example, child care grants are quite small, and only available for children under 14. More substantial government grants like the foster care grant are not available to support temporary fostering arrangements or poor parents trying to raise children within the family. Substantial foster care grants are intended only for orphans and children in the permanent care of foster parents (Meintjes et al. 2003). This inequity links into the broader debate about whether interventions should be externally driven because communities are not coping (Nyambedha et al. 2003), for example by establishing orphanages, or whether interventions should be aimed at strengthening existing community systems to cope better (Chirwa 2002).

There are compelling reasons for not singling out possibly stigmatised groups such as AIDS-affected children or orphans for interventions, especially when the cause of their disadvantage is neither AIDS nor orphanhood, but is another problem experienced in common with other children. Even where the cause of disadvantage might be AIDS or orphanhood, where the solution to the problem is the same as solutions offered to other children, there is no need to offer specific interventions for AIDS-affected children or orphans.

Researchers on AIDS and children know, however, that the reasons for children's disadvantage are not uniform, that they are not all due to orphanhood, AIDS or poverty, and that they should not all be addressed in the same way. This diversity has also been noted in studies of child poverty (Hill & Smith 2003) and education (Ainsworth & Filmer 2002).

What should researchers say to policy-makers when they find factors that seem to be associated with specific disadvantage that may require specific interventions? Using longitudinal data, Case and Ardington (2004) have been able to show that maternal death is actually more important than poverty or paternal death in determining access to education. This finding is supported by Nyamukapa and Gregson (2005). Providing free schooling may therefore help some poor children, including orphans, to go back to school, but the situation of maternal orphans may not substantially improve.

Identifying these maternal orphans as recipients of a specific intervention may be stigmatising. What needs to be done is to establish what interventions are required, to assess their cost effectiveness in terms of the number of children who might benefit from improved schooling access, and to determine how this intervention may best be implemented, perhaps by redesigning a broader initiative to include new features. In the same way, enabling access for disabled people to public buildings is often now termed 'universal access', since people with prams and the elderly using walking sticks are often just as 'disabled' by stairs as people in a wheelchair. Designing 'universal access' requires an understanding of the various difficulties people might face in order to design the best generic solution.

4.4.2 How should stigma reduction interventions for children be designed?

Given the difficulties experienced in reducing stigma in adults, or even in measuring the efficacy of anti-stigma interventions, it is difficult to say what should be done to achieve this in children. However, it is possible to make a few points at this stage that may assist in developing appropriate anti-stigma measures for children.

In developing anti-stigma interventions for adults, the most common approach has been to increase knowledge of HIV/AIDS and reduce misconceptions about the disease. The content of HIV/AIDS-related stigma will differ across different cultural and socio-economic contexts (Deacon et al. 2005), although a recent study suggests that these differences are not so large as to require different kinds of interventions (Ogden & Nyblade 2005).

Increasing children's knowledge and dispelling myths about HIV/AIDS may reduce instrumental stigma caused by inappropriate fear of transmission. Knowledge-based interventions should be developmentally appropriate for children. Mass media, comic books and computer-based applications can be attractive to youth (el-Setouhy & Rio 2003; Lee 2005). Workshopping public health information in groups has worked well with adults (Ogden & Nyblade 2005) and could be adapted for children.

Knowledge-based interventions by themselves have however been shown to have limited effect in reducing stigma and discrimination (Brown et al. 2001). Changing children's negative attitudes towards PLWHA, including children living with HIV/AIDS, is difficult. Some benefit may be gained from programs with adults, as adult attitudes filter down to children (Cossman 2004). Although increased perception of controllability does seem to be linked to stigmatising attitudes, one intervention that successfully reduced children's perceptions of obesity as a controllable disease did not significantly reduce their stigmatising attitudes (Anesbury & Tiggemann 2000). Although it is generally accepted that using negatively-associated disease terminology can exacerbate stigma, encouraging adolescents to use less pejorative labels for schizophrenia in China did not result in less stigmatising attitudes (Chung & Chan 2004).

Health-related services and educational institutions need to address the problem of stigma and discrimination directly. Just as AIDS-related information for children can be built into broader health-related programmes (Lee 2005), so too can anti-stigma messages be built into anti-bullying, anti-racism, anti-sexism and human rights education. Lyon and Woodward (2003) show how developing successful public health programmes for HIV-positive African-American adolescents in inner-city America requires public health services to openly address the problem of stigma (for example by not using stigmatising labels for clients), and to develop skills-oriented, culturally sensitive and life-affirming programmes, as well as provide solutions to transport and childcare problems faced by clients. Wiener et al. (1993) give an outline of social considerations, including stigma and discrimination, in designing appropriate hospice care for children with HIV.

Increased knowledge about disease has been associated with greater distress in children with chronic diseases and those with terminally ill parents, so any educational intervention should be accompanied by programmes providing emotional support to these categories of children, who may not be prepared to self-identify in a public forum. Given the greater control exerted by families and institutions like schools over children's environments than is possible among adults, it may in fact be easier to provide children with focused support around stigma.

Poverty relief is increasingly being seen as an anti-stigma intervention. People working on HIV and AIDS have suggested that promoting human rights and reducing inequalities in society can reduce the effects of HIV/AIDS-related stigma (Parker & Aggleton 2003). Socio-economic rehabilitation has been used as an anti-stigma intervention for people with leprosy.

4.5   Conclusion

Developing effective anti-stigma interventions for children requires that we neither focus exclusively on OVC nor on knowledge and attitudes underlying HIV/AIDS-related stigma. It is far more important to understand in what circumstances and contexts stigma has disadvantaging effects on children, and to try and limit these negative effects without singling out AIDS-affected children for special, possibly stigmatising, treatment.

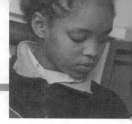

CHAPTER 5

Conclusions

In this review we have covered the key debates relevant to understanding the impact of HIV/AIDS-related stigma on children by reviewing the literature on the material and psychosocial effects of the AIDS pandemic on children, as well as the literature on children and disease-related stigma, racism and coping.

We know that HIV/AIDS-related stigma is a serious problem for infected and affected adults, reducing access to treatment, testing and care, sometimes resulting in internalisation of negative attitudes and withdrawal from social engagement by PLWHA (see Deacon et al. 2005). It is possible that stigma could be an even more serious barrier to the material and psychosocial well-being of children than it is in adults. Children could also be more vulnerable to discrimination than adults.

Compared to the huge quantity of AIDS-related stigma research on adults, there has been an under-investigation of the problem in children. Perhaps this is because even in mainstream research and interventions discourse, children have generally been seen as relatively innocent victims of the AIDS pandemic, in contrast to the way in which adults can be seen as both sexually transgressive (for example, not using condoms) and unfairly stigmatising of PLWHA. Even adolescents, who are perceived as problematic because they engage in unsafe and premature sexual activity, do not perhaps have the same power as adults to discriminate against others. However, children have now been identified as a source of both stigmatising attitudes and discriminatory behaviour (Cree et al. 2004; Letamo 2004).

Most stigma research in adults is aimed at identifying how many people stigmatise PLWHA: research on experiences of stigma is relatively new. Both children's attitudes and children's experiences of stigma have, by contrast, been under-researched. Evidence that children stigmatise each other has in fact received even less attention than evidence that children experience AIDS-related discrimination from adults. In adults, attitudes are often measured against knowledge about HIV/AIDS, partly to see whether educational interventions might help reduce stigma or discrimination. Children's knowledge about HIV/AIDS has been a focus of attention mainly in relation to prevention research and interventions, however, and not in relation to stigma. Most research attention on children has been focused on measuring the impact of the pandemic on them, especially on orphans. Stigma is mainly raised as an issue in understanding psychosocial impacts of the pandemic on children, while research on discrimination tends to focus mainly on material effects (for example, loss of inheritance, abuse, denial of care and so on).

In this paper we develop the following hypotheses to try and integrate and broaden this field of research. The hypotheses will now be discussed in turn.

5.1   Hypothesis 1: HIV/AIDS-related stigma and discrimination exacerbates the negative effects of the pandemic on children and their support systems

In general, existing research confirms that HIV/AIDS-related stigma and discrimination probably do exacerbate the effects of the pandemic on children. A number of research papers have suggested that HIV/AIDS-related stigma is a serious problem for children (Chase & Aggleton 2001; Clay et al. 2003; Geballe et al. 1995; Gernholtz & Richter 2004;

Strode & Barrett-Grant 2001). The literature on disclosure demonstrates particularly powerfully how much stigma negatively affects the lives of children infected and affected by stigmatising disease. Comparable research on epilepsy and other stigmatised diseases suggests that stigma does affect children adversely (Austin et al. 2004). Stigma, discrimination and courtesy stigma directed towards adults can also affect the ability of caregivers to provide proper psychosocial and material support for children infected or affected by HIV/AIDS (Juma et al. 2004; Robertson & Ensink 1992).

Most research on HIV/AIDS-related stigma and children focuses on a few isolated issues, such as the psychosocial effects of bereavement or disclosure; on identifying cases of discrimination for human rights advocacy; or on identifying knowledge gaps and attitudes to AIDS that could result in risk behaviours. Stigma can however have both material and psychosocial effects on children and that can have indirect effects on children through their caregivers.

Also, the effects of HIV/AIDS-related stigma on children need to be differentiated from other negative effects of the pandemic on children. We noted in Chapter 2 that all discrimination is not caused by HIV/AIDS-related stigma, so it is important to be very clear as to the cause of discrimination if one is to link it to HIV/AIDS stigma. Simply measuring disadvantage is not a proxy for measuring the effects of discrimination, nor is it a proxy for measuring the effects of stigma. Disadvantage for a stigmatised group (such as AIDS orphans) is not therefore necessarily a sign of HIV/AIDS-related stigma.

Most of the quantitative research on the effects of the pandemic on children compares the situation of orphans and non-orphans, and some studies compare AIDS orphans to other orphans, or non-orphans. AIDS-related stigma can however affect not only AIDS orphans, but children whose parents or relatives are sick with AIDS, or children who are themselves HIV-positive. Coupled with the paucity of the more detailed disclosure and parenting research in Africa, this makes it difficult to extrapolate directly from existing data in assessing the impact of HIV/AIDS-related stigma on children in sub-Saharan Africa.

5.2 Hypothesis 2: HIV/AIDS-related stigma towards children is framed within different social discourses

In exploring the effects of HIV/AIDS-related stigma on children, it is critical to understand the content and social context of stigmatising discourses. Adolescents tend to be stigmatised in relation to having HIV/AIDS mainly because of the assumption that they have contracted it through sexual activity. Younger children (whether infected or affected) tend to be stigmatised for an association with HIV/AIDS that is either framed around their parents' sexual behaviour or their own poverty or lack of a caregiver (for example, as street children or orphans). These very different forms of HIV/AIDS-related stigmatisation interact with and draw on other forms of stigma – for example, stigma around early sexual debut or promiscuity in women, around poverty itself, or around abandoned or rejected children. They may also have different meanings and effects in different contexts. What the research suggests is that it is important to research and understand stigmatising discourses around children within their social context, instead of simply measuring stigmatising attitudes on standard attitudinal scales.

5.3 Hypothesis 3: Children stigmatise each other

Children can be very cruel to each other. This can have serious and negative effects on their well-being and even on their access to education. Children's choice of stigma content also seems to be highly gendered, specific attention being paid to the status of the mother. Children tend to take familial insults very personally, so the effects of these insults may be more serious than in adults. In examining the few studies that compare children's responses to those of adults on attitudinal surveys, the jury is still out on whether children and young adults stigmatise more or less than do adults. We still do not fully understand the relationship between knowledge acquisition and attitudes. Also, problems in assessing children's attitudes through fixed-format questions may discredit the results of surveys comparing children and adults.

5.4 Hypothesis 4: Children experience HIV/AIDS-related stigma differently depending on their stage of emotional and cognitive development

In order to understand the impact of stigma on children, we need to recognise that the same stigmatising or discriminatory environment may have different effects on children depending on their stage of cognitive and emotional development, as well as other factors. Identifying these factors can inform data collection and analysis in research studies, and research that controls for such factors can help design better, more targeted interventions.

The coping literature can inform our understanding of how children cope differently with stigma at different ages. Understanding and measuring knowledge acquisition in children is very challenging, and there is no clear relationship between ignorance and stigma. Although there are some protective effects of age in dealing with stressors, the greater knowledge, insight and vulnerability to peer opinion that usually comes with age, and the greater stigmatisation of HIV infection associated with sexual activity, tend to disadvantage adolescents both in being recipients of, and in coping with, AIDS-related stigma. Younger children affected by HIV/AIDS may, however, be more likely to experience stigma and discrimination as normal and as personal,[21] and may therefore be vulnerable to internalisation of stigma. Other factors such as the actual experience of AIDS-related illness and gendered expectations of children's roles in families need to be explored in order to fully understand the differential experience of stigma by children.

5.5 What new research is needed?

In conclusion, more research is required to understand the negative effects of HIV/AIDS-related stigma on children. Research should be carefully designed to address regionalised, gendered, age-related and content-related differences in patterns of stigmatisation towards and by children. Research on the effects of stigma and discrimination needs to address material and psychosocial effects as well as direct and indirect effects. Such research needs to investigate children's knowledge and attitudes, experiences of stigmatisation, internalisation of stigma and expected stigma and discrimination as well as stigmatisation by children.

There are problems with using adult stigma scales and adult-oriented research methods to measure stigma in children. At the very least, survey instruments should be tailored towards younger children's needs by providing more concrete situations for discussion,

---

21 L Cluver, comments on this paper.

using pictures and dolls as prompts. Children's own views should be determined through self-report, but semi-structured interviews and open-ended questions with probes for underlying information and non-verbal cues should be chosen over self-report questionnaires and fixed-format questions. Researchers should attempt to gather both quantitative and qualitative data using reasonably large sample sizes, and where possible use longitudinal study designs.

In the absence of an easy definition of which children are going to be most affected by HIV/AIDS, and in areas where most children will be affected in some way, it may be pointless to search for a traditional control group. Even if we could find a control group, simply comparing the situation of affected and less affected children in cross-sectional study designs is not going to definitively identify the reasons for disadvantage. A better approach may be to collect enough data on individual children to understand degrees of vulnerability. Researchers can then analyse datasets comparing vulnerability factors and other mitigating and mediating factors against stigma measures in order to understand whether stigma increases vulnerability, and in what ways it does so.

5.6   What are the implications for interventions?

Interventions should not further stigmatise children infected or affected by HIV/AIDS, nor should they unduly privilege one group over another where problems are shared. Instead, we need to develop interventions based on an understanding of what disadvantaging effects stigma might have on children, how these are caused, and therefore, what issues need to be addressed in broader programmes. We can address a range of different causes of disadvantage in a holistic intervention without singling out stigmatised groups.

Developing effective anti-stigma interventions for children requires that we do not focus only on correcting knowledge and attitudes underlying HIV/AIDS-related stigma. Programmes for HIV/AIDS education should be integrated into broader life skills and health education programmes. They should be supplemented by human rights education aimed at tackling a range of issues including disease stigma, racism and sexism. Poverty relief, the establishment of support groups and rights-based advocacy programmes should also form part of anti-stigma interventions.

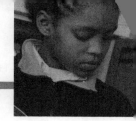

REFERENCES

Abebe T (2005) Geographical dimensions of AIDS orphanhood in sub-Saharan Africa, *Norwegian Journal of Geography* 59(1): 37–47

Aggleton P (2001) *Comparative analysis: Research studies from India and Uganda: HIV and AIDS-related discrimination, stigmatization and denial.* Geneva: UNAIDS

Ainsworth M & Filmer D (2002) *Poverty, AIDS and children's schooling: A targeting dilemma.* World Bank Policy Research Paper 2885. World Bank, Washington DC

Ali S (1998) Community perceptions of orphan care in Malawi, in *Southern African Conference on Raising the Orphan Generation*, CINDI, Pietermaritzburg

Alonzo AA & Reynolds NR (1995) Stigma, HIV and AIDS: An exploration and elaboration of a stigma trajectory, *Social Science & Medicine* 41(3): 303–315

Amon JJ (2002) Preventing HIV infections in children and adolescents in sub-Saharan Africa through integrated care and support activities: A review of the literature, *Africa Journal of Aids Research* 1(2): 143–149

Andiman W (1995) Medical aspects of AIDS: What do children witness? In Geballe S, Andiman W & Gruendel J (eds) *Forgotten children of the AIDS epidemic.* New Haven: Yale University Press

Anesbury T & Tiggemann M (2000) An attempt to reduce negative stereotyping of obesity in children by changing controllability beliefs, *Health Education Research* 15(2): 145–152

Ansell N & Young L (2004) Enabling households to support successful migration of AIDS orphans in southern Africa, *AIDS Care* 16(1): 3–10

Atwine B, Bajunirwe F & Cantor G (2005) Psychological distress among AIDS orphans in rural Uganda, *Social Science & Medicine* 61: 555–564

Austin JK, MacLeod JS, Dunn DW, Shen JS & Perkins SM (2004) Measuring stigma in children with epilepsy and their parents: Instrument development and testing, *Epilepsy & Behavior* 5(4): 472–482

Ayuku D, Odero W, Kaplan C, De Bruyn R & De Vries M (2003) Social network analysis for health and social interventions among Kenyan scavenging street children, *Health Policy and Planning* 18(1): 109–118

Baggaley R, Sulwe J, Chilala M & Mashambe C (1999) HIV stress in primary school teachers in Zambia, *Bulletin of the World Health Organization* 77(3): 284–287

Barnard M & Barlow J (2003) Discovering parental drug dependence: Silence and disclosure, *Children & Society* 17(1): 45–56

Barrett C, McKerrow N & Strode A (1999) Consultative paper on children living with HIV/AIDS: Prepared for the South African Law Commission. Wits Law Project, University of the Witwatersrand

Berger BE, Ferrans CE & Lashley FR (2001) Measuring stigma in people with HIV: psychometric assessment of the HIV stigma scale, *Research in Nursing and Health* 24(6): 518–529

Bernard C (2002) Giving voice to experiences: Parental maltreatment of black children in the context of societal racism, *Child and Family Social Work* 7(4): 239–251

Blood GW, Blood IM, Tellis GM & Gabel RM (2003) A preliminary study of self-esteem, stigma, and disclosure in adolescents who stutter, *Journal of Fluency Disorders* 28(2): 143–159

Bogart LM, Catz SL, Kelly JA, Gray-Bernhardt ML, Hartmann BR, Otto-Salaj LL, Hackl KL

& Bloom FR (2000) Psychosocial issues in the era of new AIDS treatments from the perspective of persons living with HIV, *Journal of Health Psychology* 5(4): 500–516

Boler T & Carroll K (2003) *Addressing the educational needs of orphans and vulnerable children*. UK: Save the Children and Action Aid International, UK

Bond V, Chilikwela L, Clay S, Kafuma T, Nyblade L & Bettega N (2003) *Kanayaka 'The light is on': Understanding HIV and AIDS-related stigma in urban and rural Zambia, a report*. Luaka: Zambart Project and Kara Counselling and Training Trust (KCTT)

Bond V, Ndubani P & Nyblade L (2000) Formative research on mother to child transmission of HIV/AIDS in Zambia: A working report of focus group discussions held in Keemba, Monze, November 1999. Unpublished report. Keemba MTCT Formative Research, Lusaka

Brackis-Cott E, Mellins CA & Block M (2003) Current life concerns of early adolescents and their mothers: Influence of maternal HIV, *Journal of Early Adolescence* 23(1): 51–77

Bray R 2003 Predicting the social consequences of orphanhood in South Africa, *African Journal of AIDS Research* 2(1): 39–55

Broder H & Strauss RP (1989) Self-concept of early primary school age children with visible or invisible defects, *Cleft Palate Journal* 26(2): 114–117

Brookes H, Shisana O & Richter L (2004) *The national household HIV prevalence and risk survey of South African children*. Cape Town: HSRC Press

Brown L, Trujillo L & Macintyre K (2001) *Interventions to reduce HIV/AIDS stigma: What have we learnt?* Population Council, Horizons Program Tulane University: USAID

Call KT, Riedel AA, Hein K, McLoyd V, Petersen A & Kipke M (2002) Adolescent health and well-being in the twenty-first century: A global perspective, *Journal of Research on Adolescence* 12(1): 69–98

Campbell C, Foulis CA, Maimane S & Sibiya Z (2005) 'I have an evil child at my house': Stigma and HIV/AIDS management in a South African community, *American Journal of Public Health* 95(5): 808–815

Caplan M (2002) Why are children's experiences of domestic violence being ignored? An investigation into adult resistance to helping children exposed to domestic violence. Honours thesis. University of Cape Town

Carlton-Ford S, Miller R, Nealeigh N & Sanchez N (1997) The effects of perceived stigma and psychological over-control on the behavioural problems of children with epilepsy, *Seizure* 6(5): 383–391

Case A & Ardington C (2004) *The impact of parental death on school enrolment and achievement: Longitudinal evidence from South Africa*. Working Paper No. 97. Centre for Social Science Research (CSSR), University of Cape Town

Case A, Paxson C & Ableidinger J (2003) *The education of African orphans*. Princeton: Center for Health and Well-being Research Program in Development Studies, Princeton University

Castle S (2004) Rural children's attitudes to people with HIV/AIDS in Mali: The causes of stigma, *Culture Health & Sexuality* 6(1): 1–18

Castro A & Farmer P (2005) Understanding and addressing AIDS-related stigma: From anthropological theory to clinical practice in Haiti, *American Journal of Public Health* 95(1): 53–59

Chase E & Aggleton P (2001) *Stigma, HIV/AIDS and prevention of mother-to-child transmission: A pilot study in Zambia, India, Ukraine and Burkina Faso.* UK: United Nations Children's Fund/ Panos Institute

Chatterji M, Dougherty L, Ventimigla T, Mulenga Y, Jones A, Mukaneza A, Murry N, Buek K, Winfrey W & Amon J (2005) *The well-being of children affected by HIV/AIDS in Gitarama Province, Rwanda, and Lusaka, Zambia: Findings from a study.* Working Paper No. 2. Community REACH Program, Pact, Washington D.C.

Chirwa WC (2002) Social exclusion and inclusion: Challenges to orphan care in Malawi, *Nordic Journal of African Studies* 11(1): 93–113

Chung KF & Chan JH (2004) Can a less pejorative Chinese translation for schizophrenia reduce stigma? A study of adolescents' attitudes toward people with schizophrenia, *Psychiatry and Clinical Neurosciences* 58(5): 507–515

Clacherty G (2001) *The role of stigma and discrimination in increasing vulnerability of children and youth affected by HIV/AIDS: Report on participatory workshops.* Pretoria: Save the Children UK, Pretoria.

Clacherty G & Kushlick A (2004) Meeting the challenge of research with very young children: A practical outline of methodologies used in the formative research and pre-testing of the Takalani Sesame HIV and AIDS television and radio programmes. Paper preseted at Fourth International Education Entertainment Conference, Cape Town

Claflin CJ & Barbarin OA (1991) Does 'telling' less protect more? Relationships among age, information disclosure, and what children with cancer see and feel, *Journal of Pediatric Psychology* 16(2): 169–191

Clay S, Bond V & Nyblade L (2003) *We can tell them: AIDS doesn't come through being together. Children's experiences of HIV and AIDS-related stigma in Zambia 2002–2003.* Lusaka: Zambart Project and Kara Counselling and Training Trust

Cluver L (2003) The psychological well-being of AIDS orphans in Cape Town, South Africa. Masters in Alied Social Studies, University of Oxford

Cluver L (2005) *Brief review: Quantitative research on the mental health of AIDS orphans*

Cluver L & Gardner F (in press) *Risk and protective factors for emotional well-being of orphaned children in Cape Town: A qualitative study of perspectives of children and caregivers* (submitted). Department of Social Policy and Social Work, Oxford University

Collins-Jones TL (1997) *AIDS orphans: The psychological adjustment of children with multiple family members with a terminal illness.* Dissertation Abstracts International Section B: The Sciences and Engineering 58, 2659

Connolly P (1998) *Racism, gender identities and young children: Social relations in a multi-ethnic, inner-city primary school.* London: Routledge

Consortium on Aids and International Development (2004) *Working group on orphans and vulnerable children.* UK: AIDS Consortium

Cossman JS (2004) Parents' heterosexism and children's attitudes toward people with AIDS, *Sociological Spectrum* 24(3): 319–339

Cramer JA, Westbrook LE, Devinsky O, Perrine K, Glassman MB & Camfield C (1999) Development of the quality of life in epilepsy inventory for adolescents: The QOLIE-AD-48, *Epilepsia* 40(8): 1114–1121

Crampin A, Floyd S, Glynn J, Madise N, Nyondo A, Khondowe M, Njoka C, Kanyongoloka H, Ngwira B, Zaba B & Fine P (2005) The long-term impact of HIV and orphanhood on the mortality and physical well-being of children in rural Malawi, *Aids* 17(3): 389–397

Cree VE, Kay H, Tisdall K & Wallace J (2004) Stigma and parental HIV, *Qualitative Social Work* 3(1): 7–25

Cunningham SD, Tschann J, Gurvey JE, Fortenberry JD & Ellen JM (2002) Attitudes about sexual disclosure and perceptions of stigma and shame, *Sexually Transmitted Infections* 78(5): 334

Dago-Akribi HA & Cacou Adjoua M-C (2004) Psychosexual development among HIV-positive adolescents in Abidjan, Côte d'Ivoire, *Reproductive Health Matters* 12(23): 19–28

Daileader Ruland C, Finger W, Williamson N, Tahir S, Savariaud S, Schwaitzer A-M, & Henry Shears K (2005) *Adolescents: Orphaned and vulnerable in the time of HIV/AIDS.* USA: Family Health International

Dane BO (1994) Death and bereavement. In BO Dane & C Levine (eds) *Aids and the new orphans: Coping with death.* Westport, CT: Auburn House

Dane BO & Levine C (2005) *AIDS and the new orphans: Coping with death.* Westport, CT: Auburn House

Daniel M (2005) Beyond liminality: Orphanhood and marginalisation in Botswana, *African Journal of AIDS Research* 4(3): 195–204

Davids A, Letlape L, Magome K, Makgoba S, Madivenyi C, Mdwaba T, Ned N, Nkomo N, Mfecane S & Skinner D (2006) *A situational analysis of orphans and vulnerable children in four districts of South Africa.* Cape Town: HSRC Press

De Moura SL (2004) The social distribution of reports of health-related concerns among adolescents in Sao Paulo, Brazil, *Health Education Research* 19(2): 175–184

Deacon H, Stephney I & Prosalendis S (2005) *Understanding HIV/AIDS stigma: A theoretical and methodological analysis.* Cape Town: HSRC Press

Devinsky O, Westbrook L, Cramer J, Glassman M, Perrine K & Camfield C (1999) Risk factors for poor health-related quality of life in adolescents with epilepsy, *Epilepsia* 40(12): 1715–1720

Dodge B & Khiewrord U (2005) *Coping with love: Older people and HIV/AIDS in Thailand.* UK: Help Age International

Donald P, Gosling S & Hamilton J (1995) `No problem here?' *Children's attitude to race in a mainly white area.* Edinburgh: The Scottish Council for Research in Education

Dunn DW & Austin JK (1999) Symptoms of depression in adolescents with epilepsy, *Journal of the American Academy of Child & Adolescent Psychiatry* 38(9): 1132

Eisenberg N, Fabes RA & Guthrie IK (1997) Coping with stress: The roles of regulation and development. In Wolchik SA & Sandler IN (eds) *Handbook of children's coping: Linking theory and intervention.* New York: Plenum Press

Eiser C, Havermans T, Craft A & Kernahan J (1995) Development of a measure to assess the perceived illness experience after treatment for cancer, *Archives of Disease in Childhood* 72(4) (electronic): 302–307 el-Setouhy MA & Rio F (2003) Stigma reduction and improved knowledge and attitudes towards filariasis using a comic book for children, *Journal of the Egyptian Society of Parasitology* 33(1): 55–65

Flanagan-Klygis E, Ross LF, Lantos J, Frader J & Yogev R (2002) Disclosing the diagnosis of HIV in pediatrics, *Aids & Public Policy Journal* 17(1): 3–12

Forehand R, Armistead L, Summers P, Morse S, Morse E & Clark L (1999) Understanding of HIV/AIDS among children of HIV-infected mothers: Implications for prevention, disclosure and bereavement, *Children's Health Care* 28(4): 277–295

Forehand R, Steele R, Armistead L, Morse E, Simon P & Clark L (1998) The Family Health Project: Psychosocial adjustment of children whose mothers are HIV infected, *Journal of Consulting and Clinical Psychology* 66(3): 513–520

Forehand R, Armistead L, Wierson M, Brody GH, Neighbors B & Hannan J (1997) Hemophilia and AIDS in married men: Functioning of family members – Hemophilia PAC Project, *American Journal of Orthopsychiatry* 67(3): 470–464

Forsyth BW (2003) Psychological aspects of HIV infection in children, *Child and Adolescent Psychiatric Clinics of North America* 12(3): 423–437

Foster G, Makufa C, Drew R, Mashumba S & Kambeu S (1997) Perceptions of children and community members concerning the circumstances of orphans in rural Zimbabwe, *AIDS Care* 9(4): 391–405

Foster G & Williamson J (2000) A review of current literature on the impact of HIV/AIDS on children in sub-Saharan Africa, *Aids* 14 (Sul 3): S275–S284

Fox K (2004) *Watching the English: The hidden rules of English behaviour.* London: Hodder

Fox S (2002) Hidden needs of children: Psychosocial support for children affected by HIV/AIDS. Paper presented at the 14th International Aids Conference, 7-12 July, Barcelona, Spain

Garvey M (2003) *Dying to learn: Young people, HIV and the churches - A Christian aid report*. UK: Christian Aid

Gaughan DM, Hughes MD, Oleske JM, Malee K, Gore CA, Nachman S & for the Pediatric AIDS Clinical Trials Group (2004) Psychiatric hospitalizations among children and youths with Human Immunodeficiency Virus infection, *Pediatrics* 113(6): e544-e551

Geballe S, Gruendel J & Andiman W (1995) *Forgotten children of the AIDS epidemic*. New Haven, CT: Yale University Press

Gernholtz L & Richter M (2004) Access of abandoned children and orphans with HIV/AIDS to antiretroviral therapy – a legal impasse, *South African Medical Journal* 94(11): 910–912

Gewirtz A & Gossart-Walker S (2000) Home-based treatment for children and families affected by HIV and AIDS dealing with stigma, secrecy, disclosure, and loss, *Child and Adolescent Psychiatric Clinics of North America* 9(2): 313–330

Giese S, Meintjes H & Proudlock P (2002) *National Children's Forum on HIV/AIDS, 22–24 August 2001: Workshop report*. Cape Town: Children's Institute, University of Cape Town

Giese S, Meintjes H, Croke R & Chamberlain R (2003a) The role of schools in addressing the needs of children made vulnerable in the context of HIV/AIDS. Document distributed in preparation for the Education Policy Round Table, 28–29 July 2003, Children's Institute, University of Cape Town

Giese S, Meintjes H, Croke R & Chamberlain R (2003b) Health and social services to address the needs of orphans and other vulnerable children in the context of HIV/AIDS. Research report and recommendations report submitted to HIV/AIDS directorate, National Department of Health, January 2003. Cape Town: Children's Institute, University of Cape Town

Gilborn L, Nyonyintoro R, Kabumbuli R & Jagwe-Wadda G (2001) *Making a difference for children affected by AIDS: Baseline findings from operations research in Uganda.* Washington: Horizons Program

Gomo E, Rusakaniko S, Mashange W, Mutsvangwa J, Chandiwana B & Munyati S (2006) *Household survey of HIV-prevalence and behaviour in Chimanimani District, Zimbabwe, 2005: A baseline survey.* Cape Town: HSRC Press

Goodwin RA, Kozlova A, Nizharadze G & Polyakova G (2004) HIV/AIDS among adolescents in Eastern Europe: Knowledge of HIV/AIDS, social representations of risk and sexual activity among school children and homeless adolescents in Russia, Georgia and the Ukraine, *Journal of Health Psychology* 9(3): 381–396

Gosling AS, Burns J & Hirst F (2004) Children with HIV in the UK: A longitudinal study of adaptive and cognitive functioning, *Clinical Child Psychology & Psychiatry,* 9(1): 25–37

Goulder PJ, Jeena P, Tudor-Williams G & Burchett S (2001) Paediatric HIV infection: correlates of protective immunity and global perspectives in prevention and management, *British Medical Bulletin* 58(1): 89–108

Gow J & Desmond C (2002) *Impacts and interventions – The HIV/AIDS epidemic and the children of South Africa.* Durban: University of Natal Press

Granados J, Amador S, De Miguel M, Tome P, Conejo P, Vivas JC, Pollan J, Contreras J & Espert A (2003) Impact of highly active antiretroviral therapy on the morbidity and mortality in Spanish human immunodeficiency virus-infected children, *The Pediatric Infectious Disease Journal* 22(10): 863–868

Grassly N, Lewis J, Mahy M & Walker N (2004) Comparison of household-survey estimates with projections of mortality and orphan numbers in sub-Saharan Africa in the era of HIV/AIDS, *Population Studies* 58(2): 207–217

Grassly NC & Timaeus IM (2003) *Orphans and AIDS in sub-Saharan Africa.* New York: United Nations

Green SE (2003) What do you mean 'what's wrong with her?': Stigma and the lives of families of children with disabilities, *Social Science & Medicine* 57(8): 1361–1374

Green SE, Davis C, Straight B, Karshmer E & Marsh P (2005) Living stigma: The impact of labeling, stereotyping, separation, status loss, and discrimination in the lives of individuals with disabilities and their families, *Sociological Inquiry* 75(2): 197–215

Greene PJ (1980) The doll technique and racial attitudes, *Pacific Sociological Review* 23(4): 474–490

Hackl KL, Somlai AM, Kelly JA & Kalichman SC (1997) Women living with HIV/AIDS: The dual challenge of being a patient and caregiver, *Health and Social Work* 22(1): 53–62

Hamra M, Ross MW, Karuri K, Orrs M & D'Agostino A (2005) The relationship between expressed HIV/AIDS-related stigma and beliefs and knowledge about care and support of people living with AIDS in families caring for HIV-infected children in Kenya, *AIDS Care-Psychological and Socio-Medical Aspects of AIDS/HIV* 17(7): 911–922

Harrington R & Harrison L (1999) Unproven assumptions about the impact of bereavement on children, *Journal of the Royal Society of Medicine* 92(5): 230–233

Harvey RD (2001) Individual differences in the phenomenological impact of social stigma, *Journal of Social Psychology* 141(2): 174–189

Herek GM (2002) Thinking about AIDS and stigma: A psychologist's perspective, *Journal of Law Medicine & Ethics* 30(4): 594

Heywood M (2002) Chaffed and waxed sufficient: Drug access, patents and global health, *Third World Quarterly, Journal of Emerging Areas* 23(2): 1–19

Hill S & Smith C (2003) Creating the real picture – Child well-being and poverty indicators in South Africa: Report of the workshop held in Cape Town and the establishment of a Child Research Network. SARPN, South Africa

Hinshaw SP (2004) Parental mental disorder and children's functioning: Silence and communication, stigma and resilience, *Journal of Clinical Child and Adolescent Psychology (formerly Journal of Clinical Child Psychology)* 33(2): 400–411

Hirsch WM (2001) *A comparison between AIDS-orphaned children and other-orphaned children on measures of attachment security and disturbance,* Dissertations Abstracts International, 61(11-B): 6137

Hough ES, Brumitt G, Templin T, Saltz E & Mood D (2003) A model of mother-child coping and adjustment to HIV, *Social Science & Medicine* 56(3): 643–655

Ingram D & Hutchinson SA (1999) HIV-positive mothers and stigma, *Health Care for Women International* 20(1): 93–103

International HIV/AIDS Alliance (2003) *Building blocks in practice – Africa-wide briefing notes: Social inclusion.* UK: International HIV/AIDS Alliance

International HIV/AIDS Alliance & Help Age International (2004) *Building blocks: Africa-wide briefing notes: Supporting older carers.* UK: Help Age International

Jeena PM, McNally LM, Stobie M, Coovadia HM, Adhikari MA & Petros AJ (2005) Challenges in the provision of ICU services to HIV infected children in resource poor settings: A South African case study, *Journal of Medical Ethics* 31(4): 226–230

Joffe H & Bettega N (2003) Social representation of AIDS among Zambian adolescents, *Journal of Health Psychology* 8(5): 616–631

Joffe H (1999) *Risk and 'The other'.* Cambridge: Cambridge University Press

John K & Sainsbury C (2003) *The impact of HIV/AIDS on older people in Cambodia.* UK: Help Age International

Johnson SR, Schonfeld DJ, Siegel D, Krasnovsky FM, Boyce JC, Saliba PA, Boyce WT & Perrin EC (1994) What do minority elementary school students understand about the causes of acquired immunodeficiency syndrome, colds, and obesity? *Journal of Developmental and Behavioral Pediatrics* 15(4): 239–247

Juma M, Okeyo T & Kidenda G (2004) '*Our hearts are willing, but*'. *Challenges of elderly caregivers in rural Kenya*. Nairobi: Population Council

Kaaya SF, Mukoma W, Flisher AJ & Kle KI (2002) School-based sexual health interventions in sub-Saharan Africa: A review, *Social Dynamics* 28(1): 64–88

Kalichman SC & Simbayi LC (2003) HIV testing attitudes, AIDS stigma, and voluntary HIV counselling and testing in a black township in Cape Town, South Africa, *Sexually Transmitted Infections* 79(6): 442–447

Kamali A, Seeley JA, Nunn JA, Kengeya-Kayondo JF, Ruberantwari A & Mulder DW (1996) The orphan problem: experience of a sub-Saharan Africa rural population in the AIDS epidemic, *AIDS Care* 8(5): 509–515

Kelly K & Ntlabati P (2002) Early adolescent sex in South Africa: HIV intervention challenges, *Social Dynamics* 28(1): 42–63

Khongkunthian P, Grote M, Isaratanan W, Piyaworawong S & Reichart PA (2001) Oral manifestations in 45 HIV-positive children from Northern Thailand, *Journal of Oral Pathology and Medicine* 30(9): 549–552

Kmita G, Baranska M & Niemiec T (2002) Psychosocial intervention in the process of empowering families living with children living with HIV/AIDS – a descriptive study, *AIDS Care* 14(2): 279–284

Koerner SS, Wallace S, Lehman SJ & Raymond M (2002) Mother-to-daughter disclosure after divorce: A double-edged sword? *Journal of Child and Family Studies* 11: 496-483

Krasnik A & Wangel M (1990) AIDS and Danish adolescents – knowledge, attitudes, and behaviour relevant to the prevention of HIV-infection, *Danish medical bulletin* 37(3): 275–279

Krener P & Miller FB (1989) Psychiatric response to HIV spectrum disease in children and adolescents, *Journal of the American Academy of Child and Adolescent Psychiatry* 28(4): 596–605

Laas S (2004) *The psychosocial adjustment of adolescent AIDS orphans: Internalizing and externalizing difficulties*. Cape Town: University of Cape Town

Leclerc-Madlala S (2002) Youth, HIV/AIDS and the importance of sexual culture and context, *Social Dynamics* 28(1): 20–41

Lee K (2005) *The Pulse pilot evaluation report 2005*. UK: The African Pulse

Lee MB & Rotheram-Borus MJ (2002) Parents' disclosure of HIV to their children, *Aids* 16(16): 2201–2207

Lee MY (2001) Marital violence: Impact on children's emotional experiences, emotional regulation and behaviors in a post-divorce/separation situation, *Child and Adolescent Social Work Journal* 18(2): 137–163

Leslie MB, Stein JA & Rotheram-Borus MJ (2002) The impact of coping strategies, personal relationships, and emotional distress on health-related outcomes of parents living with HIV or AIDS, *Journal of Social and Personal Relationships* 19(1): 45–66

Lester P, Chesney M, Cooke M, Whalley P, Perez B, Petru A, Dorenbaum A & Wara D (2002) Diagnostic disclosure to HIV-infected children: How parents decide when and what to tell, *Clinical Child Psychology and Psychiatry* 7(1): 85–99

Letamo G (2003) Prevalence of, and factors associated with, HIV/AIDS-related stigma and discriminatory attitudes in Botswana, *Journal of Health, Population and Nutrition* 21(4): 347–357

Letamo G (2004) HIV/AIDS-related stigma and discrimination among adolescents in Botswana, *African Population Studies* 1–14

Letteney S & Laporte HH (2004) Deconstructing stigma: Perceptions of HIV-seropositive mothers and their disclosure to children, *Social Work in Health Care* 38(3): 105–123

Lewis E (2001) *Afraid to say: The needs and views of young people living with HIV/AIDS*. London: National Child's Bureau Enterprises Ltd

Lichtenstein B, Laska MK & Clair JM (2002) Chronic sorrow in the HIV-positive patient: issues of race, gender, and social support, *AIDS Patient Care STDS* 16(1): 27–38

Lim VK, Teo TS, Teo AC & Tan KT (1999) HIV and youths in Singapore – knowledge, attitudes and willingness to work with HIV-infected persons, *Singapore Medical Journal* 40(6): 410–415

Lindblade KA, Odhiambo F, Rosen DH & Decock KM (2003) Health and nutritional status of orphans < 6 years old cared for by relatives in western Kenya, *Tropical Medicine & International Health* 8(1): 67–72

Link BG & Phelan JC (2001) Conceptualizing stigma, *Annual Review of Sociology* 27(1): 363–385

Link BG & Phelan JC (2006) Stigma and its public health implications, *Lancet* 367(9509): 528–529

Lipson M (1994) Disclosure of diagnosis to children with human immunodeficiency virus or acquired immunodeficiency syndrome, *Journal of Developmental and Behavioral Pediatrics* 15(3): S61–S65

Lobato D, Barbour L, Hall LJ & Miller CT (1987) Psychosocial characteristics of preschool siblings of handicapped and non-handicapped children, *Journal of Abnormal Child Psychology (Historical Archive)* 15(3): 329–338

Lutzke JR, Ayers TS, Sandler IN & Barr A (1997) Risks and interventions for the parentally bereaved child. In S Wolchik & IN Sandler (eds) *Handbook of children's coping: Linking theory and intervention*. New York: Plenum Press

Lyon ME & Woodward K (2003) Nonstigmatizing ways to engage HIV-positive African-American teens in mental health and suort services: A commentary, *Journal of the National Medical Association* 95(3): 196–200

Macklin R (1992) Autonomy, beneficence, and child development: An ethical analysis. In B Stanley & JE Sieber (eds) *Social research on children and adolescents: Ethical issues*. Sage Publications

MacLeod JS & Austin JK (2003) Stigma in the lives of adolescents with epilepsy: A review of the literature, *Epilepsy & Behavior* 4(2): 112

Madhavan S (2004) Fosterage patterns in the age of AIDS: Continuity and change, *Social Science & Medicine* 58(7): 1443–1454

Mahati ST, Chandiwana B, Munyati S, Chitiyo G, Mashange W, Chibatamoto P & Mupambireyi PF (2006) *A qualitative assessment of orphans and vulnerable children in two Zimbabwean districts*. Cape Town: HSRC Press

Makame V, Ani C & Grantham-McGregor S (2002) Psychological well-being of orphans in Dar El Salaam, Tanzania, *Acta Paediatrica* 91(4): 459–465

Mathews C, Guttmacher SJ, Flisher AJ, Mtshinzana Y, Hani A & Zwarenstein M (2005) Written parental consent in school-based HIV/AIDS prevention research, *American Journal of Public Health* 95: 1266–1269

Mawn B (1999) Raising a child with HIV: An emerging phenomenon, *Families, Systems & Health* 17(2): 197–215

Meintjes H, Budlender D, Giese S & Johnson L (2003) *Children 'in need of care' or in need of cash? Questioning social security provisions for orphans in the context of the South African AIDS pandemic.* Cape Town: Children's Institute, Centre for Actuarial Research, University of Cape Town

Meintjes H & Giese S (2006) *Spinning the epidemic: The making of mythologies of orphanhood in the context of AIDS.* Cape Town: Children's Institute and Centre for Social Science Research, University of Cape Town

Melvin D, Krechevsky D & Divac A (2005) Parental reports of the incidence of emotional and behavioural difficulties in HIV-infected school-age children using the Goodman strengths and difficulties screening measure: Initial findings from a multi-centre study in London. In *Psychology, Health and Medicine* 12(1): 40-47

Michielutte R & Diseker RA (1982) Children's perceptions of cancer in comparison to other chronic illnesses, *Journal of Chronic Disease* 35(11): 843–852

Miles R (1989) *Racism.* London: Routledge

Mills E (2004) *Beyond the disease of discrimination: A critical analysis of HIV-related stigma in KTC, Cape Town.* CSSR Working Paper No. 100. Centre for Social Science Research, University of Cape Town

Monasch R & Boerma JT (2004) Orphanhood and childcare patterns in sub-Saharan Africa: An analysis of national surveys from 40 countries, *Aids* 18(Sul 2): S55–S65

Mturi AJ & Nzimande N (2003) *HIV/AIDS and child labour in South Africa: A rapid assessment The case study of KwaZulu-Natal.* Geneva, Switzerland: International Labour Organisation

Mukumbira R (2002) *Shock treatment for widows as pandemic ravages Zimbabwe.* African News, Nairobi, Kenya: Koinonia Media Centre

Muller O, Sen G & Nsubuga A (1999) HIV/AIDS, orphans, and access to school education in a community of Kampala, Uganda, *AIDS (London, England)* 13(1): 146–147

Murphy DA, Roberts KJ & Hoffman D (2002) Stigma and ostracism associated with HIV/AIDS: Children carrying the secret of their mothers' HIV+ serostatus, *Journal of Child & Family Studies* 11(2): 191–202

Nagler SF, Adnopoz J & Forsyth BWC (1995) Uncertainty, stigma and secrecy: Psychological aspects of AIDS for children and adolescents. In Geballe S, Gruendel J & Andiman W (eds) *Forgotten children of the AIDS epidemic.* New Haven: Yale University Press

Nampanya-Serpell N (1999) *Children orphaned by HIV/AIDS in Zambia: Risk factors from premature parental death and policy implications.* PhD Thesis, University of Maryland, Baltimore

Nattrass N (2002) AIDS and human security in Southern Africa, *Social Dynamics* 28(1): 1–19

Nehring WM, Lashley FR & Malm K (2000) Disclosing the diagnosis of pediatric HIV infection: Mothers' views, *Journal of the Society of Pediatric Nurses* 5(1): 5–14

Nelkin D & Gilman SL (1988) Placing blame for devastating disease, *Social Research* 55(3): 361–378

Nelms BC (1989) Emotional behaviors in chronically ill children, *Journal of Abnormal Child Psychology (Historical Archive)* 17(6): 657–668

Newell ML, Brahmbhatt H & Ghys PD (2004) Child mortality and HIV infection in Africa: A review, *Aids* 18: S27–S34

Ntozi JPM & Mukiza-Gapere J (1995) Care for Aids orphans in Uganda: Findings from a focus group discussion, *Health Transition Review* 5(Suppl. 2): 245–252

Nyambedha EO, Wandibba S & Aagaard-Hansen J (2003) Changing patterns of orphan care due to the HIV epidemic in western Kenya, *Social Science & Medicine*, 57(2): 301–311

Nyamukapa C & Gregson S (2005) Extended family's and women's roles in safeguarding orphans' education in AIDS-afflicted rural Zimbabwe, *Social Science & Medicine* 60(10): 2155–2167

O'Hare BAM, Venables J, Nalubeg JF, Nakakeeto M, Kibirige M & Southall DP (2005) Home-based care for orphaned children infected with HIV/AIDS in Uganda, *AIDS Care* 17(4): 443–450

Obeidallah D, Turner P, Iannotti RJ, O'Brien RW, Haynie D & Galper D (1993) Investigating children's knowledge and understanding of AIDS, *The Journal of School Health* 63(3): 125–129

Ogden J & Nyblade L (2005) *Common at its core: HIV-related stigma across contexts.* Washington DC: International Center for Research on Women

Ostrom RA, Serovich JM, Lim JY & Mason TL (2006) The role of stigma in reasons for HIV disclosure and non-disclosure to children, *AIDS Care* 18(1): 60–65

Parker R & Aggleton P (2003) HIV and AIDS-related stigma and discrimination: A conceptual framework and implications for action, *Social Science & Medicine* 57(1): 13–24

Pattman R & Chege F (2003) 'Dear diary I saw an angel, she looked like heaven on earth': Sex talk and sex education, *African Journal of AIDS Research* 2(2): 103–112

Pawinski R & Lalloo U (2001) Community attitudes to HIV/AIDS, *South African Medical Journal* 91(6): 448

Paxton S (2002) The paradox of public HIV disclosure, *AIDS Care* 14(4): 559–567

Peltzer K & Promtussananon S (2003) Black South African children's understanding of health and illness: Colds, chicken pox, broken arms and AIDS, *Child Care Health and Development* 29(5): 385–393

Percy A, McAlister S, Higgins K, McCrystal P & Thornton M (2005) Response consistency in young adolescents' drug use self-reports: A recanting rate analysis, *Addiction* 100(2): 189–196

Pfeffer CR, Karus D, Siegel K & Jiang H (2000) Child survivors of parental death from cancer or suicide: depressive and behavioral outcomes, *Psychooncology* 9(1): 1–10

Poindexter CC (2002) 'It don't matter what people say as long as I love you': Experiencing stigma when raising an HIV-infected grandchild, *Journal of Mental Health and Aging* 8(4): 331–348

Policy Project, Centre for the Study of AIDS, USAID, & Department of Health (2003) *Siyam'kela: Measuring HIV/AIDS related stigma: A report on the fieldwork.* Cape Town: Policy Project

Poulter C (1997) *A psychological and physical needs profile of families living with HIV/AIDS in Lusaka, Zambia.* Research Brief 2. UNICEF, Lusaka

Prior L, Wood F, Lewis G & Pill R (2003) Stigma alone does not explain non-disclosure of psychological symptoms in general practice, *Evidence-Based Mental Health* 6(4): 128

Pugatch D, Bennett L & Patterson D (2002) HIV medication adherence in adolescents: A qualitative study, *Journal of HIV/AIDS Prevention & Education for Adolescents & Children* 5(1): 9–29

Rebhun LA (2004) Sexuality, color, and stigma among Northeast Brazilian women, *Medical Anthropology Quarterly* 18(2): 183–199

Reyland SA, Higgins-D'Alessandro A & McMahon TJ (2002) Tell them you love them because you never know when things could change: Voices of adolescents living with HIV-positive mothers, *AIDS Care* 14(2): 285–294

Richter L, Manegold J & Pather R (2004) *Family and community interventions for children affected by AIDS.* Cape Town: HSRC Press

Ritsher JB, Otilingam PG & Grajales M (2003) Internalized stigma of mental illness: psychometric properties of a new measure, *Psychiatry Research* 121(1): 31–49

Robertson BA & Ensink K (1992) The psychosocial impact of human immunodeficiency virus infections in children, *Southern African Journal of Child and Adolescent Psychiatry* 4(2); 46–49

Ross MW & Rosser BR (1996) Measurement and correlates of internalized homophobia: a factor analytic study, *Journal of Clinical Psychology* 52(1): 15–21

Rotheram-Borus MJ, Weiss R, Alber S & Lester P (2005) Adolescent adjustment before and after HIV-related parental death, *Journal of Consulting and Clinical Psychology* 73(2): 221–228

Sandler IN, Tein JY & West SG (1994) Coping, stress, and the psychological symptoms of children of divorce: A cross-sectional and longitudinal study, *Child Development* 65: 1744–1763

Santana MA & Dancy BL (2000) The stigma of being named AIDS carriers on Haitian-American women, *Health Care Women International* 21(3): 161–171

Save the Children Alliance (2005) *Mitigation of HIV / AIDS impact on orphans, vulnerable children and their families.* Chimuara and Caia Baseline Study: An annex to the Save the Children Overall Baseline Study, London: Save the Children Alliance and Hope for African Children Initiative (HACI)

Schenk K & Williamson J (2005) *Ethical approaches to gathering information from children and adolescents in international settings: Guidelines and resources.* Washington DC: Horizons/Population Council

Schonfeld DJ (1997) Informing children of their human immunodeficiency virus infection, *Archives of Pediatrics & Adolescent Medicine* 151(10): 976–977

Segu M & Wolde-Yohannes S (2000) *A mounting crisis: Children orphaned by HIV/AIDS in sem-iurban Ethiopia*. Orphan Alert: International Perspectives on Children Left Behind by HIV/AIDS, Boston: François-Xavier Bagnoud Foundation

Sengendo J & Nambi J (1997) The psychological effect of orphanhood: A study of orphans in Rakai district, *Health Transition Review: The Cultural, Social, And Behavioural Determinants Of Health* 7 (Suppl): 105–124

Siegel K & Gorey E (1994) Childhood bereavement due to parental death from AIDS, *Journal of Developmental and Behavioral Pediatrics* 15(3): 66–70

Siegel K, Karus D & Raveis V (1996) Adjustment of children facing the death of a parent due to cancer, *Journal of the American Academy of Child and Adolescent Psychiatry* 35(4): 442–450

Silver Pozen A (1995) HIV/AIDS in the school. In Boyd-Franklin N, Steiner GL & Boland MG (eds) *Children, families, and HIV/AIDS*. USA: Guilford Press

Simbayi L, Kleintjes S, Ngomane T, Tabane CEM, Mfecane S & Davids A (2006) *Psychological issues affecting orphaned and vulnerable children in two South African communities*. Cape Town: HSRC Press

Skinner D (2002) Stigma and the ABCD: A consideration in South Africa. Paper read at the African Conference on the Social Aspects of HIV/AIDS Research, Promoting an African Alliance to mitigate the impact of the epidemic in Southern Africa. Pretoria: HSRC 1-4 September

Skinner D, Tsheko N, Mtero-Munyati S, Segwabe M, Chibatamoto P, Mfecane S, Chandiwana B, Nkomo N, Tlou S & Chitiyo G (2004) *Defining orphaned and vulnerable children*. Cape Town: HSRC Press

Smart R (2003) *Policies for orphans and vulnerable children: A framework for moving ahead*. Washington DC: POLICY Project, USAID

Stats SA (Statistics South Africa) (2005) *Mid-year population estimates, South Africa 2005*. Pretoria: Statistics South Africa

Stein J (1996) Coping with HIV infection: The theory and the practice, *African Anthropology III*: 2

Stein J (2003a) *Sorrow makes children of us all: A literature review on the psychosocial Impact of HIV/AIDS on children*. CSSR Working Paper No. 4. Centre for Social Science Research, University of Cape Town

Stein J (2003b) HIV/AIDS stigma: The latest dirty secret, *African Journal of AIDS Research* 2(2): 95–101

Stein JA, Riedel M & Rotheram-Borus MJ (1999) Parentification and its impact on adolescent children of parents with AIDS, *Family Process* 38(2): 193–208

Strode A & Barrett-Grant K (2001) *The role of stigma and discrimination in increasing vulnerability of children and youth infected with and affected with HIV/AIDS*. UK: Save the Children

Swart-Krueger J & Richter LM (1997) AIDS-related knowledge, attitudes and behaviour among South African street youth: Reflections on power, sexuality and the autonomous self, *Social Science & Medicine (1982)* 45(6): 957–966

Tanzania Stigma-Indicators Field Test Group (2005) *Measuring HIV stigma: Results of a field test in Tanzania.* Washington DC: USAID

UNAIDS, UNICEF & USAID (2004) *Children on the brink 2004: A joint report of new orphan estimates and a framework for action.* New York: USAID

Urassa M, Boerma JT, Ng'weshemi JZL, Isingo R, Schapink D, Kumogola Y, Awusabo-Asare K, Pisani E & Zaba B (1997) Orphanhood, child fostering and the AIDS epidemic in rural Tanzania, *Health Transition Review* 7(Suppl. 2): 141–153

Valente SM (2003) Depression and HIV disease, *JANAC: Journal of the Association of Nurses in AIDS Care* 14(2): 41–51

Vallerand AH, Hough E, Pittiglio L & Marvicsin D (2005) The process of disclosing HIV serostatus between HIV-positive mothers and their HIV-negative children, *Aids Patient Care and Stds* 19(2): 100–109

Van Ausdale D & Feagin JR (2001) *The first R: How children learn race and racism.* Boston Way, Lanham: Rowman & Littlefield Publishers

Wailoo K (2001) Stigma, race, and disease in twentieth century America, *The Lancet* 367: 531-33

Watney S (1996) 'Risk groups' or 'risk behaviors?' In J Mann & D Tarantola (eds) *AIDS in the World II.* New York: Oxford University Press

Webb D (1995) Who will take care of the AIDS orphans? *AIDS Analysis Africa* 5(2): 12–13

Weisberg LA & Ross W (1989) AIDS dementia complex: Characteristics of a unique aspect of HIV infection, *PostgradMed* 86(1): 213–220

West A & Wedgwood K (2004) Children affected by Aids, orphans, and impact mitigation in China. In *Third Asia Public Policy Workshop and the Fourth WHR Rivers Symposium Social Development, Social Policy and HIVAIDS in China,* Harvard University 6-8 May

Wiener LS, Battles HB, Heilman N, Sigelman CK & Pizzo PA (1996) Factors associated with disclosure of diagnosis to children with HIV/AIDS, *Pediatric AIDS and HIV Infection* 7(5): 310–324

Wiener L, Fair C & Pizzo PA (1993) Care for the child with HIV infection and AIDS Care for the child with HIV infection and AIDS. In Armstrong-Dailey A & Goltzer SZ (eds) *Hospice care for children.* New York: Oxford University Press

Wiener LS, Battles HB & Heilman N (2000) Public disclosure of a child's HIV infection: Impact on children and families, *AIDS Patient Care & STDs* 14(9): 485–497

Wild L (2001) The psychosocial adjustment of children orphaned by AIDS, *Southern African Journal of Child and Adolescent Mental Health* 13(1): 3–22

Wild LG, Flisher AJ, Laas S & Robertson BA (2005) The psychosocial adjustment of adolescents orphaned in the context of HIV/AIDS. (Draft.) University of Cape Town

Wolchik S & Sandler IN (1997) *Handbook of children's coping: Linking theory and intervention.* New York: Plenum Press

Worsham NL, Compas BE & Ey S (1997) Children's coping with parental illness. In SA Wolchik & IN Sandler (eds) *Handbook of children's coping: Linking theory and intervention.* New York: Plenum Press

Young B, Dixon-Woods M, Windridge KC & Heney D (2003) Managing communication with young people who have a potentially life threatening chronic illness: Qualitative study of patients and parents, *British Medical Journal* 326(7384): 305–310

Zickmund S, Ho EY, Masuda M, Iolito L & LaBrecque DR (2003) 'They treated me like a leper' - Stigmatization and the quality of life of patients with hepatitis C, *Journal of General Internal Medicine* 18(10): 835–844

Zuyderduin JR (2004) The buddy system of support and care for and by women living with HIV/AIDS in Bostwana. Doctoral Thesis, University of South Africa